HEALING PLANTS

Self-treatment of the most common everyday complaints
and disorders with selected medicinal plants. Time-tested
recipes for teas, tea blends, tinctures, ointments, inhalations,
compresses, and baths. Expert advice and dependable remedies.

GUIDE TO PROPER TREATMENT

Self-treatment with Healing Plants

Medicinal plants are time-tested natural medicines. Like all other medicinal preparations, however, they can have undesirable side effects along with curative effects. Treatment of complaints and disorders with medicinal plants can be successful only if the right plants are used in a selective way, and if the limits of their applicability are observed conscientiously.

If you would like to treat yourself with medicinal plants, please follow these four rules—then you can use these plants responsibly, and you will be assured of safety in your self-treatment.

1 Evaluate Your Complaints Properly

In this manual, 11 groups of complaints are described clearly in separate chapters. Use the table of contents to choose the chapter that applies to you. The index (see page 218) also will help you find the proper application. Please read the comments on your complaints with great care and discuss them with your physician. You will learn to evaluate your problems correctly and determine whether self-treatment is possible or sensible.

2 Select the Application Carefully

The clearly outlined complaints are followed in every instance by the appropriate applications of healing plants.

If several different formulations are recommended for treating a complaint, try them individually to see which one helps you most.

The length of treatment is also noted. The compendium of medicinal plants (see page 137) will provide you with valuable information on your favorite herbs.

3 Prepare and Administer the Application as Directed

Many of the healing plant applications suggested in this book can be put into effect by following a uniform set of directions for preparation and usage. You will find standard directions for the applications on pages 216–217. Any divergent instructions are given in the text where appropriate. Please follow these directions exactly.

4 Observe the Limits of Self-treatment

We wish to emphasize that you bear sole responsibility when under treatment. Before starting, therefore, please note the remarks on page 7, The Limits of Self-treatment. The efficacy of medicinal plant applications is described clearly, as are potential problems that may occur during the treatment. Nevertheless, we strongly suggest that you discuss your condition and your intended treatment with your physician.

In addition, note the special warnings given at appropriate places in the text.

Important Note

In this large Barron's manual, the use of medicinal plant applications to treat the most common everyday complaints and disorders is described. Readers must assume full responsibility for deciding whether and to what extent they wish to use medicinal plants in treating their ailments.

● Please pay close attention to the warnings in the text and to the comments on The Limits of Self-treatment.

● Please inform your physician of your intention to treat yourself with healing plants.

Contents

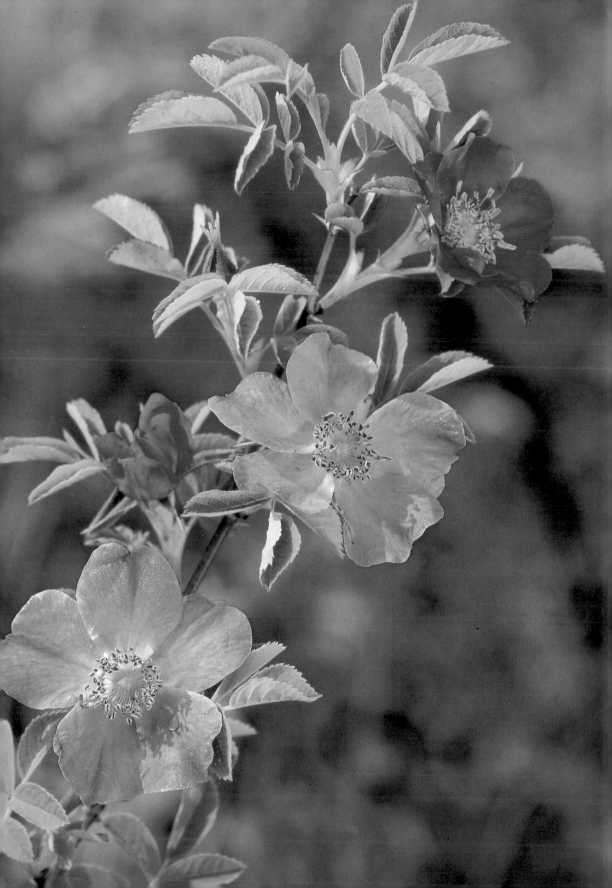

Self-help with Healing Plants

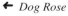 *Dog Rose*

Preface

Medicinal plants have quite an eventful history: At one time they were the only healing agents known to us; knowledge of their effects was passed on from one generation to the next. The pharmaceutical-botanists and the physician-botanists of antiquity were the first, followed by the monks in the Middle Ages, to make a written record of their empirical knowledge. In their works many of these authors made important statements—in some cases still valid today—about the healing effects of plants.

The development of herbal medicine suffered a brief setback around 1600, when new remedies—chemical compounds—were introduced. Nevertheless, people retained their confidence in the healing powers of plants. With the invention of printing, herbals found wide distribution. In the sixteenth and seventeenth centuries there appeared the works of Leonhard Fuchs, Hieronymus Bock, and Petrus Andreas Matthiolus—names still familiar to specialists in medicinal plants. In the United States, John Uri Lloyd (1849–1936) and Heber W. Youngken, Sr. (1885–1963), gave fresh impetus to the study of pharmacognosy and botanical medicine.

Since that time, pharmacognosy, the study of medicinal plants as a source of therapy, and phytotherapy, the branch of knowledge dealing with the use of medicinal plants, have become sciences. The substances contained in plants are being identified and their effects are being researched. Explanations are being found for what we once knew only through experience.

We can no longer imagine medicine without medicinal plants; it is precisely the most successful medicaments that frequently contain active substances derived from plants.

Nevertheless, in the 1950s, medicinal plants once again were briefly pushed into the background by chemical preparations. Because they take effect swiftly, these preparations also often were used indiscriminately to treat everyday complaints, but they often did more harm than good.

After all, anything that has an effect also has side effects! The faster and more powerfully an agent takes effect, the greater can be the side effects. Consequently, people once again recalled the healing powers of time-tested officinal herbs.

In this renaissance of medicinal plants, however, something essential was overlooked, at least at the beginning: the limits of their applicability! Medicinal plants were indiscriminately celebrated as remedies "from God's pharmacy," and their use was recommended irresponsibly, even for cases in which they accomplish nothing. Medicinal plants can bring about cures, and they can have palliative and preventive effects—but they are not miracle drugs. Phytotherapy can be successful only if the right medicinal plants are employed to good purpose and the limits of their applicability are observed scrupulously—particularly in a course of self-treatment.

In this large Barron's guide to healing plants I provide you with information on responsible ways of self-treatment with preparations derived from medicinal plants—teas, tinctures, baths, inhalations, compresses, poultices, and washes. For these purposes I have selected primarily those medicinal plants that have been subjected to extensive scientific research, recognized as possessing therapeutic effects, and—in most cases—approved as natural medicines by the German Office of Health; that is, medicinal plants that can be relied upon. [Note: The listings of the German Office of Health (Bundesgesundheitsamt) are generally regarded as the most authoritative in the world. Ed.]

In this book I give you directions for treating the most common everyday disorders and aches and pains, including severe and chronic problems. I offer relief for anyone suffering from rheumatism and gout, bladder and kidney trouble, colds, nervousness and sleep disturbances, gastric and intestinal complaints, and gallbladder and liver disorders, as well as minor injuries, skin irritations, and wounds.

I have devoted special attention to childhood diseases, as children are not "little adults"; they often have to be treated differently. Older people also will find remedies for their special ailments in this book. It is a book for all those who want to stay fit and healthy with medicinal plant applications or who want to regain their health quickly, but it also is intended for people who want to use medicinal plants appropriately in support of a physician's therapy—a book, in short, that a health-conscious family can use daily. So that you can treat yourself successfully, I have tried to answer all the questions that might arise.

Please read carefully the directions for the correct preparation of the medicinal plant applications, particularly the teas (see page 14). It is absolutely essential to follow the dosage instructions (see page 14); otherwise, the medicinal plants will not have the desired effect.

To preserve the quality of the drugs—the dried medicinal plants—it is necessary to store them properly. I have listed everything you need to know about storage (see page 12).

The guide to proper treatment (see page 14) will lead you quickly to the application appropriate for you.

Keep this in mind: Medicinal plants are not cure-alls! For this reason you need to adhere precisely to the limits of self-treatment. To make this easier for you, I have provided both general guidelines (see opposite column) and special warnings that accompany the individual groups of disorders. For your own protection, you must follow these guidelines.

To give you greater familiarity with the efficacious medicinal plants that I have recommended for your use, I have compiled the most important information about them in the Compendium of Medicinal Plants (see page 137): their appearance, blooming season, time of harvesting, habitat, and active substances, along with their often colorful history.

If you plan to lay out a little garden of medicinal plants or if you want to cultivate your favorites in an existing garden or raise them in balcony and patio tubs, you also will find the necessary information in that chapter, under the heading Cultivation.

I hope this book will serve you and your family as a dependable guide.

The Limits of Self-treatment

We now know that medicinal plants occasionally have substantial side effects. If improperly used, employed in excessive doses, or taken for overly long periods, they can do sick people more harm than good. Only medicinal plants that have been selected with deliberation, properly prepared, and administered in the proper doses are remedies.

In the self-treatment of any complaint, therefore, responsibility for your own actions is a prime necessity. In concrete terms, this means that it is advisable to discuss your intentions with your family doctor—not least, in order to get a correct diagnosis.

If you want to treat (supposedly) harmless aches and pains without asking your doctor because you have experience in dealing with medicinal plants, here is my advice: If the problems do not disappear after three days at most, or if they reappear soon after you stop drinking the tea, then a doctor must be consulted. Severe pain and high fever are alarm signals that also require a visit to the doctor. *If, after you use the medicinal plants, other problems such as stomachache, nausea, vomiting, or diarrhea occur, or if allergic skin changes appear, discontinue the applications at once and—if the problems don't disappear quickly (after about two days)— seek a physician's advice without fail.*

It probably goes without saying that pregnant women or people with organic diseases must not treat themselves. In chronic illnesses, applications of medicinal plants can be quite beneficial as an adjunct therapy, in addition to the measures prescribed by the physician.

> **Please note**
> To keep treatment with medicinal plants from degenerating into quackery, please respect the limits of the application scrupulously; above all, also note the guidelines in the individual chapters!

What You Need to Know About Medicinal Plants

How Do Medicinal Plants Act?

In earlier times precious little thought was given to the underlying causes of the effectiveness of medicinal plants. On the basis of experience accumulated and passed on by many generations, it was known that certain plants were able to alleviate the symptoms of a great many diseases and disorders and to assist in the healing process. People relied on this body of experiential knowledge—they were forced to do so, because it was not yet possible to conduct a scientific investigation of the plants and their therapeutic effects.

Today we no longer have to make do with nothing more than our ancestors' experience; we now know why medicinal plants are such valuable remedies. With the aid of modern scientific methods, the substances contained in each plant can be isolated, analyzed, and tested for their effect. An enormous number of substances have been detected in the cells and cell sap of our medicinal plants: effective and (apparently) ineffective ones, sometimes in large quantities, sometimes only in traces. Gradually scientists succeeded in determining definitively which medicinal plants are effective and which are unsuitable. The significance of a medicinal plant, however, should not be based solely on the kinds and amounts of active substances found in them; the "little," "inconspicuous" accompanying substances in a medicinal plant also have a decisive influence on its effect. Medicinal plants are not merely vehicles for active substances; they are healing power in herbal form. The typical action of a medicinal plant is synergistic, based on the totality of all the substances it contains. Nevertheless, some groups of these substances, which are of interest not only to scientists, play a significant role in assessing the effect of the medicinal plants. You can find additional information on this subject in the following section, Medicinal Plants and the Substances They Contain.

Many medicinal plants lend themselves to the treatment of multiple diseases and conditions—that is what makes them so special. Elderberry flower tea, for example, is a time-tested sudorific (sweat-inducing agent) and cold remedy; however, this tea also alleviates rheumatic pain. Thyme lessens the irritation of dry coughs and whooping cough, but it also is effective against diarrhea and flatulence. All teas brewed from medicinal plants activate overall body metabolism by providing mild healing stimuli.

Medicinal plants are effective, and whatever has an effect can also have side effects. For this reason I have to warn you explicitly not to arbitrarily declare a medicinal herbal tea your "house tea," that is, to drink it in large quantities over a long period.

A course of treatment that involves drinking an herbal tea regularly for longer than six to eight weeks has to be discussed with your physician. Often, however, the complaints will disappear after only a few days. In most cases they are gone after two or three weeks.

Medicinal Plants and the Substances They Contain

Active Substances—Nonparticipating Substances
The active substances in medicinal plants are substances that a plant has produced and stored in itself during its growth. Not all of these metabolic products, however, are of direct pharmaceutical value. Active substances and neutral substances exist side by side in every medicinal plant. The neutral substances, also known as nonparticipating or inert substances, often regulate the effectiveness of the herbal healing agent by speeding up or slowing down the absorption of the substances into the organism.

A medicinal plant almost always contains several pharmaceutically effective substances, one of which—the primary active substance—determines the plant's medicinal use. How strongly the secondary active substances influence the action of a medicinal plant becomes clear when the primary active substance is isolated. Then it often has a different effect. It is the interplay among all the substances, including the neutral ones, that lends a medicinal plant its specific effect. The active substances in a medicinal plant are not distributed evenly throughout the plant. Sometimes they are stored in greater concentrations in the flowers, leaves, or roots, sometimes in the seeds, fruits, or bark.

The amount of active substances in a medicinal plant fluctuates; it is determined by the plant's habitat and by the harvesting and preparation. By harvesting at the proper time and exercising extreme care in processing, you can largely prevent problems caused by variations in strength. High quality medicinal plants are available in some pharmacies and health food stores (herb shops). Well-prepared medicinal plants, if properly stored, lose little of their effectiveness even in the drying process.

A great many medicinal plants reach maximum effectiveness only when used over a long period of time (a tea drunk regularly for six or eight weeks, for example). Use the Index to locate precise details along with the individual recipes for herbal teas.

The term "drug" is used here for dried, expertly processed medicinal plants or their parts. Pharmacists have always used the word "drug" to refer to dried medicinal plants; "druggist," the term used to designate a professional pharmacist in some countries, is derived from it. Only quite recently did "drug" also become generally accepted to denote habit-forming substances of various kinds.

To gain a better understanding of the substances and their action, it is helpful to become more familiar with the major groups of active substances contained in our medicinal plants. Here it is not so much the chemical composition that matters, but the degree of efficacy against certain ailments. In addition to the groups of active substances listed below, medicinal plants also contain substances that mean little to a layman but can give important clues to an expert.

No attempt has been made to give a general explanation because of the complicated composition (chemical structure) and the equally complicated mechanism of action.

Bitter Constituents

There are a great many plants that contain bitter-tasting substances. When we speak here of bitter-constituent drugs, however, we mean only those medicinal plants whose operative principle can be attributed solely to the presence of so-called "bitters."

Bitter-constituent drugs are called *Amara* in phytotherapy. Subdividing them as follows has proved helpful:
● Pure bitters; *Amara tonica*.
● Bitters that contain, along with the bitter constituents, a significant quantity of essential oil and therefore have a bitter, aromatic taste; *Amara aromatica*.
● Bitters that also contain acrid substances or essential oil and therefore have a bitter, acrid taste or a bitter, aromatic taste; *Amara acria* or *Acria aromatica*.

There are a great many medicinal plants that are classified as pure bitters, *Amara tonica*, but a smaller, more manageable number of these have gained wide recognition and can be recommended as particularly effective. Bitter constituents powerfully stimulate the secretion of gastric juice and, moreover, display a tonic (strengthening) overall effect. For this reason, bitter-constituent drugs can be used successfully to treat lack of appetite and to improve digestion. They are particularly helpful in dealing with various debilities: Convalescents and people suffering from anemia and nervous exhaustion will find a sure remedy in a course of treatment with bitter-constituent drugs. Typical drugs in this category are European centaury and gentian.

Bitter-constituent drugs that simultaneously contain essential oil, that is, the *Amara aromatica*, do not differ substantially in their effect from the pure bitters, the *Amara tonica*, but they contribute an additional factor—the effect of the essential oils, which extends their range of applicability. Wormwood and yarrow are important representatives of this group. In general, this can be said about the effect of the *Amara aromatica*: They act on the stomach in the same way as the bitter-constituent drugs with the addition of essential oils. Often this effect is heightened, because the scent of the essential oils stimulates the secretion of gastric juice in a reflex process. Their action, however, also extends to the intestines and influences gallbladder and liver function. Because essential oils have an antiseptic (bactericidal) effect, the *Amara aromatica* also acquire a certain antibacterial and antiparasitic effect. If fermentation is occurring in the intestinal tract, the broader influence of these drugs is especially valuable. In addition, some of them are slightly diuretic, and this side effect usually is quite welcome.

Bitters that contain acrid substances and therefore taste bitter and acrid, i.e., *Amara acria*, include ginger, for example. These drugs improve circulatory function. The effect of the bitter constituents is supported here by the acrid substances.

Dr. Hans Glatzl, an internist and a professor of nutritional physiology, determined that digestion places greater stress on the circulatory system than was previously assumed. The bitter-constituent drugs *Amara tonica, Amara aromatica,* and, in particular, *Amara acria* can counteract this strain on the circulation.

Essential Oils

Essential or volatile oils are also known as ethereal oils, but despite the "ether" component of this word, such oils have nothing to do with the ether that previously was used as an anesthetic.

The essential oils contained in plants are by nature highly volatile substances, but in water they are only sparingly soluble or completely insoluble. They smell acrid and, with few exceptions, unpleasant. Essential oils are common in the plant kingdom; few plants are completely free of these oils. In botanical medicine, however, only those medicinal plants that have an especially high content of these "scented oils"—0.1 to 10 percent—are classified as essential-oil drugs. These include especially the representatives of two botanical families, the Lamiaceae (Labiatae) and the Apiaceae (Umbelliferae). Within the plant, the essential oils are stored in special "oil containers," the oil cells, oil ducts,

or oil glandular hairs. Essential oils are composed of a great many diverse substances. In a single essential oil, over 100 separate substances were identified.

The medicinal plants that contain essential oils have the following therapeutic effects in common: They are anti-inflammatory in cases of more or less severe skin irritation; expectorant (facilitating the expulsion of phlegm from the respiratory tract); diuretic; antispasmodic; and tonic (strengthening) for the stomach, intestinal tract, gallbladder, and liver. Drugs with essential oils combat fermentative agents (zymogens), bacteria, and possibly even viruses. Here, however, we have to understand clearly that "combat" is not synonymous with "destroy completely."

Flavonoids

The word "flavonoid" (flavone) is a collective term for various substances with the same basic chemical structure. It is difficult to characterize the action of the flavonoid-containing drugs, because the kinds and amounts of flavonoids they contain are the determining factors. Flavonoids have extremely diverse chemical and physical properties, and for this reason no single consistent effect can be assumed to exist. Nevertheless, several effects are typical: an effect on abnormal capillary fragility; an effect on certain cardiac and circulatory disorders; a diuretic and antispasmodic effect on the digestive tract. Without doubt, flavonoids frequently play an active role in the overall effect of a medicinal plant.

Tannins

Tannins, in the pharmaceutical sense, are plant substances that are able to bind proteins of the skin and the mucous membranes and transform them into resistant, insoluble substances. Their therapeutic effect is based on this: they deprive the bacteria that have settled on the skin or mucosae of their nutritive medium. They may also inactivate bacteria directly. We know and use some medicinal plants that contain tannins as their primary active substance (for example, erect cinquefoil, also known as tormentil or bloodwort, and blueberries), other plants in which tannin is present as a welcome secondary active substance, and still others in which the tannin has an unpleasant effect, as it can irritate the stomach (for example, bearberry leaves). If you don't want to avoid the third category, prepare the teas by the cold-water method; then only a fraction of the tannins will make their way into the tea.

Tannin drugs stand us in good stead as a gargle for sore throats, a mouthwash for inflamed gums, a compress for wounds, and, above all, a means to combat diarrhea. Similarly, partial baths with tannin drugs are recommended therapeutic measures for hemorrhoids, frostbite, and inflammations.

Some medicinal plants contain tannins that may inactivate certain prescription and over-the-counter (OTC) drugs. Therefore, it is advisable to ingest medicinal plant remedies either one hour before or two hours after prescription or OTC drugs are taken orally.

Glycosides

Glycosides are substances that occur widely throughout the plant kingdom. Their effects are so numerous and so diverse that the use of a single chemical term—glycosides—to include all of them actually tells us little: It all depends on the effects. The term "glycoside drugs," however, has become a fixture in the scientific literature and appears here for that reason. All glycosides have a common feature: They can be split by hydrolysis (decomposition of a compound into other compounds by taking up water) into a sugar and a non-sugar, the aglycone. The aglycone largely determines the effect. Examples of glycosides are the substances found in some medicinal plants that act as cardiac stimulants and expectorants, the laxative substances of alder buckthorn bark, and the active substances of bearberry leaves.

The sudorific, or sweat-causing, effect of linden flowers and the effect of many bitter-constituent drugs are also attributable to glycosides.

Silicic Acids

Plants from the horsetail (Equisetaceae), borage (Boraginaceae), and grass (Poaceae or Gramineae) families absorb a great deal of silicic acid from the ground and store it in their cell membranes or cell substance (protoplasm). In many cases the salts of silicic acid (silicates) are water-soluble. Because silicic acid is also an essential component of the human organism, silicic acid drugs can be used to bring about improvement where a decrease in the supply of this acid in the diet has resulted in damage, particularly to connective tissue, skin, hair, or nails.

A drug in frequent pharmaceutic use is field horsetail, which is taken internally in the form of tea and used externally as a gargle, mouthwash, and bath additive.

Saponins

Saponins are surface active herbal glycosides that, when shaken with water, produce long-lasting froth and foam and that emulsify oil in water. They have a hemolytic effect; that is, they cause the hemoglobin to escape when added to a suspension of red blood cells. Saponin drugs can be used to treat stubborn coughs. The surface activity of the saponins causes the viscid mucus to liquefy, and the phlegm can be coughed up more easily.

The mucus newly produced by the body can drain freely. There is a slight stimulating effect upon the gastric mucous membranes, and in a reflex process the secretion of all the glands increases, which brings about improvement inside the bronchial tubes.

Many saponin drugs also have a diuretic effect and are frequently called upon for use in so-called blood-purifying, (depurative), treatments (in spring and fall).

They also are effective against skin blemishes and rheumatic complaints. Moreover, many saponin drugs can reputedly decrease edemas and act as anti-inflammatories. Not least, saponins in medicinal plants can decisively influence the resorption of other active plant substances, so that minute quantities of active substances often have a "big" effect. Saponins are not entirely harmless, however—an excess will irritate the intestinal mucous membranes.

Mucilage

Mucilage in the botanical and pharmacological sense refers to carbohydrate-containing substances that expand greatly when mixed with water and produce a viscous (stringy) liquid. Mucilage drugs are widespread in the plant kingdom, but only a few plants—marshmallow, flax, and Iceland moss, for example—contain amounts sufficient for therapeutic use. In many other instances, however, they have a decisive influence on the intensity of the effects of other active plant substances. The pharmacological effect of plant mucilage can best be described as "soothing, lessening irritation."

When ingested, a thin layer coats the mucous membranes and thus protects them against local irritants or reduces the irritation. Inflammations, particularly those affecting the mucous membranes, subside quickly under the influence of mucilage drugs. Mucilage is not absorbed, so the effect is purely local. Mucilage drugs can have a cough-relieving, or antitussive, effect if the cough is caused by irritating conditions in the throat and on the epiglottis. Some mucilage drugs are slightly laxative because they loosen the contents of the bowels, retain water, and expand (flaxseed, or linseed). One particular characteristic of mucilage is the ability to lessen the sensation of taste, especially where sour substances are concerned. An impressive example: Raspberries contain less sugar and more acids than red currants, but because their mucilage content is higher, they taste sweeter than red currants.

Vitamins, Minerals, and Trace Elements

The so-called essential nutrients have to be included in any presentation of the most important substances contained in plants. They are needed in the organism to build the ingredients of its framework (connective tissue, bones, teeth) and cell structures; to supply building blocks for endogenous enzymes; to activate metabolic processes; and to influence organ functions and water balance. Without these sub-

stances, life is utterly impossible. An ample, well-balanced supply of them in the diet is vital. This explains the significance of foods of plant origin in our diet (vegetables, salad, fruits). In the treatment of diseases where a deficiency of minerals, trace elements, and vitamins is present, preparations made from medicinal plants containing these substances are particularly important. Minerals, trace elements, and vitamins are partially dissolved when an infusion of tea is prepared, and thus they also have a part to play in the therapeutic effect. If a certain vitamin is the primary active substance of a medicinal plant, the drug can be employed to good purpose as a supplier of vitamins. This applies, for example, to rose hips, which are extremely rich in vitamin C.

Storing Medicinal Plants Correctly

Always store dried medicinal herbs in opaque glass containers or in tins. They will be protected from light, dampness, and insects, and will better retain their quality.

The labeling of the storage containers is also important, as dried and crushed medicinal plants—the tea drugs—are difficult to tell apart. In addition, put in the container a slip of paper noting the date on which you bought the plant or prepared one you collected yourself, the name of the family member who was treated with the tea, the problems that were treated successfully, and the dose that proved helpful.

At one time most pharmacies could furnish medicinal herbs, but this service has diminished over the last 25 years. However, in view of the recent interest in "natural medicines," many pharmacies now provide common medicinal plants; health food stores are excellent sources.

Weighing, Mixing, and Measuring Plant Substances

You may purchase balances (scales) for weighing out the ingredients for the tea blends or single herbs recommended in this guide. After being weighed, each ingredient should be crushed or broken between the fingers or in a mortar and pestle to the coarseness, if possible, of a black tea-cut (i.e., open a tea bag to observe the relative size of the material). All ingredients should be mixed thoroughly. This is carried out most easily by placing all the crushed ingredients into a small paper bag and shaking thoroughly to ensure a uniform mixture.

For measuring liquids (small quantities) it is convenient to use a 100 milliliter graduated cylinder or pharmaceutical graduate from your pharmacist.

The number given with the various recipes represent ounces/grams or fluid ounces/milliliters. For example, .70/20 = .70 ounces/20 grams of chamomile; .35/10 = .35 fluid ounces/10 milliliters of tincture of valerian.

Should You Collect Medicinal Plants Yourself?

If you want to collect some medicinal plants yourself, you absolutely must have extensive knowledge of botany. You can test the adequacy of your knowledge relatively easily. Just ask yourself these questions:

● Can I recognize unerringly the medicinal plant I'm looking for when I see it in the wild?
● Do I know that some medicinal plants have poisonous "doubles?"
● Do I know which medicinal plants are poisonous and hence unsuitable for self-medication because they are highly dangerous?
● Do I know which medicinal plants are on the list of protected plants and may not be collected under any circumstances?
● Do I know in what kind of environment I can collect medicinal plants—can I tell whether a meadow, a field, or the edge of a forest is free of environmental pollution?
● Do I know at what time of day and in what season I should gather the medicinal plant of my choice to maximize its effectiveness?

● Do I know which part of the plant is used as a "drug" for making tea—the flowers, fruits, seeds, roots, bark, or all the aerial parts?
● Do I know how to prepare properly all the plants I gather? If the answer is yes, do I have the opportunity to do so?

Please note
If the root is the part to be used, collecting is out of the question; you would endanger the wild population of the medicinal plant! Roots used for medicinal purposes (also for teas) are specially cultivated.

If this "examination of your conscience" has revealed that you know little about medicinal plants, for the time being you should make no attempt to collect them yourself.

If this guide has aroused your interest, however, and you would like to learn more, you can add to your knowledge by reading reliable books on medicinal plants and guides to collecting plants (see Books for Further Reading, page 224).

You can grow some of the medicinal plants mentioned in this book in your own garden or as tub plants on your balcony or patio. You will learn how to raise them in the Compendium of Medicinal Plants (see page 137) under the heading Cultivation.

Self-treatment

Preparation and Application of the Teas

Herbal teas are medicinal preparations. Like other medicines, they are most effective when they are used purposefully and in the correct doses. Preparing teas according to directions is also of great importance: The amount used, the water temperature, the length of the steeping time, and even the method of drinking the tea (in sips, warm, hot, or cold) are significant. For all these reasons, please follow the exact instructions in this book, so that the tea can be fully effective.

To make dealing with medicinal herbal teas easier for you, I have tried to find a uniform method of preparation for most of the teas recommended in this book.

The following directions apply, unless other instructions are given in the specific recommendations for each tea:

Preparation of the teas:
Pour 8 ounces (1/4 L) of boiling water over 2 heaping tablespoonfuls of the drug (a single tea or a tea blend), let steep, covered, for ten minutes, then strain.

Internal Application of the Teas:
● Usual dose:
Between meals, drink two to three cups of moderately warm tea in sips. You can sweeten the tea with honey, unless you are diabetic.

Please follow equally conscientiously any other instructions that appear in the text!

External Application of the Teas:
In addition to internal application—drinking tea—you also can use medicinal teas externally; this is true of unblended teas in particular. External application refers to using tea as a gargle, mouthwash, or eyewash or to massage one's gums, treat wounds, or prepare steam baths, enemas, compresses, and full or partial baths.

● **Full baths:**
Take full baths with drug extracts in your bathtub at temperatures between 95 and 100.4°F (35–38°C) for periods of about 10 to 15 minutes. Bed rest is recommended afterward, as the warmth of the bed intensifies the aftereffect of the bath. Medicinal bath extracts based on plants are available in pharmacies and herbal shops. There is an advantage to using these ready-made extracts, because it is somewhat tedious to prepare the herbal extract for a bath yourself. Nevertheless, wherever herbal baths are recommended in the text I have also given directions for making extracts at home.

● **Partial baths:**
Partial baths for soaking injured limbs (finger, hand, foot) are quite simple: Prepare a tea and soak the afflicted parts of your body in it at a moderate temperature (95 to 104°F [35–40°C]) for about ten minutes. You need 1 tablespoonful of the drug per quart (1 L) of water. Pour the cold water over the tea, bring it to a boil, let it steep for ten minutes, strain it, and let it cool to the prescribed temperature.

● **Progressively hot footbaths:**
An important application for warding off incipient colds is the footbath in water at increasing temperatures. It results in a thorough warming of the entire body, stimulates circulation in the mucous membranes of the nose, and stops an incipient cold, a viral infection, in its tracks, because temperatures above 100.4°F (38°C) do not agree with the pathogens.

For the bath you will need a deep footbath and warm to hot water. In the footbath place 1 quart (1 L) of thyme tea (*Preparation*, see page 14) and 1 pint (1/2 L) of horsetail tea (*Preparation*, see page 14). Begin your footbath with the water at 98.6°F (37°C). Increase the temperature slowly by adding hot water as long as the heat is bearable. Stop after about 10 to 15 minutes, dry your feet, and put on warm socks.

● **Inhalations and steam baths:**
Place a small handful of tea herbs in a pot and cover with 1 pint to 1 quart (1/2–1 L) of boiling

water. For the inhalation, cover your head and the container with a cloth and inhale the herbal vapors, breathing slowly and deeply through your mouth and/or nose.

For the steam bath, allow the vapors to act on your skin. If the steam stops rising, the liquid has to be reheated to "revive" it, as the treatment should last about five to ten minutes.

For steam baths to treat the anal or genital areas, you need a stable container (a metal or porcelain bucket) on which you can sit. You will need 3 quarts (3 L) of liquid to start with and 3 to 4 tablespoonfuls of herbs.

● **Compresses:**
For damp dressings or wound compresses, soak a cotton or gauze pad in the tea, squeeze it out slightly, and place it on the areas to be treated. The compress should remain in place for several hours; the dressing, until dry. To keep the dressing damp without having to replace it, you can moisten it frequently with more of the tea if it dries out.

● **Washes:**
For herbal tea washes (highly recommended for treating skin blemishes), dip a clean cloth or piece of gauze into the lukewarm tea and, with circular motions, wash the affected areas of skin. If your goal is to remove crusts of blood, secretions, or pus, first soak a piece of gauze in the tea (as hot as you can bear) and press it on the encrusted areas. After ten minutes, begin the cleaning process. By then the crusts will be softened, and they can be washed off painlessly.

● **Gargle and mouthwash:**
For gargling and rinsing out your mouth, use the normal herbal tea—unsweetened, of course. The important thing is that the treatment be sufficiently long. The actual gargling time (minus the necessary interruptions) should total at least one minute, and the rinsing of your mouth should last about five minutes.

● **Eye compresses:**
The recommended tea, *unsweetened*, may also be used to prepare soothing eye compresses as follows. Dip a cotton pad or piece of gauze into the filtered, warm tea (not too hot). Close the eye(s) and place the wet compress on the eyelid allowing it to remain there for three to five minutes. Do not permit the tea to get into the eye. If desired, the compress may be re-dipped and re-applied. Finally, when finished, the eyelid should be patted dry with clean cotton or gauze.

● **Herbal bags:**
They can be used to soften, bring to a head, or open swellings or to alleviate pain with their heat. For this reason, herbal bags should be quite warm to hot when applied; the temperature is determined by what is bearable. Put the drug into a small linen bag and place it in boiling-hot water for about ten minutes. Let it drip dry and cool slightly, then lay it on the afflicted area.

Please note
If you have diseased veins or cardiac and circulatory problems, you should not take a hot footbath unless your physician expressly gives you permission.

If you have not already done so, please read The Limits of Self-treatment on page 7.

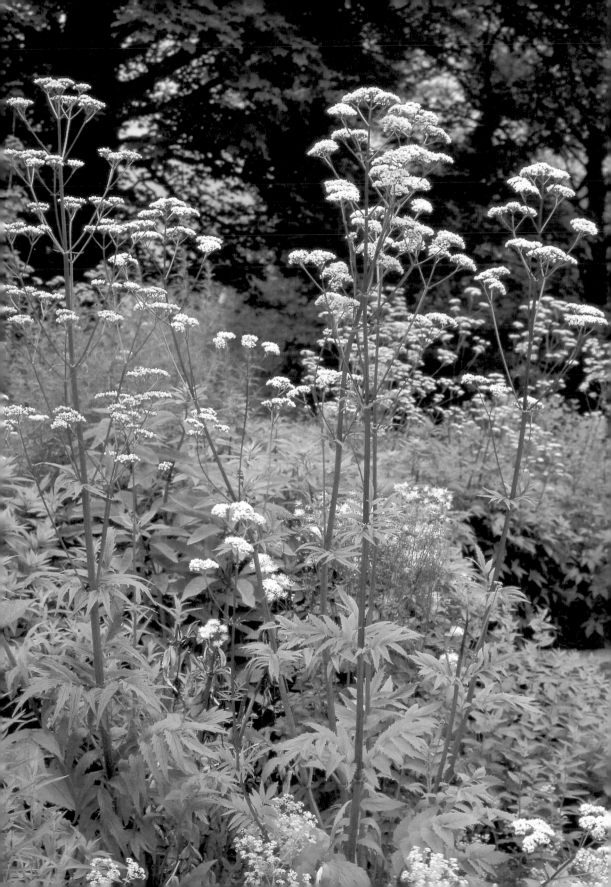

Nervousness and Sleep Disturbances

← *Valerian*

Excessive Strain Resulting from Stress

Many medicinal plants that we use today to combat nervousness, stress, and sleep disturbances were already known in olden times, though their fields of application frequently were different.

Valerian, for example, has been used as a sedative only since the nineteenth century. In the fifth and fourth centuries B.C. it was used chiefly for gynecological problems; in the Middle Ages (sixteenth to seventeenth centuries) it was a remedy for headache, coughs, or visual disturbances.

An oil made from St. John's wort previously was used largely in the treatment of wounds. Only now has it become valued primarily as a medicinal plant that has a calming effect on the psyche.

For this reason, a question suggests itself: Is nervousness a symptom of our times? Earlier times were anything but peaceful and leisurely, it is true, but people coped more easily with their problems. Everyone had his or her place in society; everyone knew what to do and what not to do; this gave people a certain confidence in their behavior, a certain "stability" within their sphere of life.

The fact is that today more and more people cannot handle their everyday life: Decline in performance, lack of drive, irritability, nervousness, difficulty going to sleep or sleeping through the night, anxieties, and joylessness are the consequences. "Stress" is the catchword, and a sense of being under stress—that is, overburdened—is common to blue-collar and white-collar workers alike, to managers and politicians, housewives and mothers, trainees, college students, even school children (see page 97). They all want help. "There must be something that can help me!" "Is there really no remedy for it?" These and similar questions are heard repeatedly.

Help from Medicinal Plants

I am in no way trying to claim that all problems can be solved with teas made from medicinal herbs. Quite often another therapy is necessary! Medicinal plants can be valuable in treating the symptoms of stress, however, because they ease tensions and create a sense of equilibrium, thereby opening the door again to the joy of living and laughter. "Merriment," according to Arthur Schopenhauer, "is a characteristic that makes us happy most directly and is its own instantaneous reward."

If we succeed in finding rest and relaxation after a job well done, then we also can better manage the stress to which we all are exposed to in varying degrees.

Over a period of many years, I have found my own favorites among the medicinal plants that have a calming and relaxing effect.

For the most part, these are well-tried medicinal plants like valerian, lemon balm, hop, chamomile, or St. John's wort. Some, such as passionflower or orange flowers, are less well known, and others—oats and lavender flowers, or hayseed—have been rediscovered.

I understand and use them all as mediators and helpers to promote a sense of well-being and balance without causing any physical or mental harm. Proper employment of them, individually or in tea blends, is of prime necessity in achieving success. I would like to pass on to you my experiences, accumulated over years of using these medicinal plants.

Symptoms and Their Treatment

"What a day; I don't want to see or hear anything else today; I'm not hungry either." Many people utter these or similar complaints in the evening: The office worker who was "hauled over the coals" by the boss, possibly without having deserved it; the individual who still has to do housework after a day in the office; the mother whose children wanted one thing after another of her all day or, even worse, are sick;

the teacher who couldn't manage the class; the businessperson who had to satisfy some difficult customers. Any number of examples can be cited. Even children often feel "unbearably stressed" (see page 98).

In such situations, anyone who swallows his or her anger will scarcely be able to sleep; the next day will be even harder to get through, and sleep again will not come easily—a vicious cycle. Finally, such people may end up with stomach trouble, often even with stomach ulcers, or their heart and circulatory system may be impaired.

Anger

● **Lemon balm tea**
You need to relax, disengage, and recover! Warm, strong tea made from lemon balm leaves is the best first-aid measure.

Preparation: Pour 8 ounces (1/4 L) of boiling water over 2 heaping teaspoonfuls of lemon balm leaves, let steep for ten minutes, then strain.

Application: Drink two to three cups of tea daily. If you like, sweeten it with honey (diabetics should not sweeten it).

Lemon balm tea is also beneficial if the day's anger has upset your stomach, because the essential oil in the lemon balm calms a nervous stomach.

Lack of Appetite

● **Lemon balm tea with hop**
If you have no appetite, you can increase the effectiveness of lemon balm tea by adding hop. In addition to calming substances, the cone-like hop fruits also contain bitter constituents, which improve the flow of gastric juice. The result is a noticeable increase in appetite.

Preparation: Pour 8 ounces (1/4 L) of boiling water over 2 heaping teaspoonfuls of lemon balm leaves and 1/2 teaspoonful of hop cones (called strobiles), let steep for five minutes, then

strain. Please do not sweeten this tea; its ability to stimulate the appetite would be impaired.

Application: Drink two to three cups of tea daily.

Stomach Trouble

● **Chamomile tea**
The third medicinal plant used to allay excessive tension resulting from stress is the wild chamomile. If your stomach is acting up because anger resulted in an excess of acid, a single cup of chamomile tea can bring release from tension. Chamomile tea calms the irritated nerves of the stomach and stops the nonphysiological (unnatural) production of acid.

Preparation and application, see page 14.

It is worth your while to experiment a bit with these three medicinal plants to find out which single tea or which tea blend is your best release from tension.

Exhaustion

● **Tea blend**
If you want rapid benefits from a tea because you are too exhausted to look much longer for a remedy, you can find rest and relief of tension, sleep and recovery in a sedative and soporific tea that I recommend adding to your household medicine chest. This tea is also suitable for use in a course of treatment to stabilize your nerves and help you sleep better over the long run:

	oz. (g)
St. John's wort, aerial parts	.70 (20)
Lemon balm leaves	.67 (19)
Raspberry leaves	.45 (13)
Hawthorn leaves and flowers	.38 (11)
Peppermint leaves	.35 (10)
Valerian roots	.24 (7)
Hop cones	.24 (7)
Passionflower, aerial parts	.24 (7)
Lavender flower	.21 (6)

Preparation: Pour one cup of boiling water over 1 heaping teaspoonful of this blend, let steep for three to five minutes, then strain. Sweetening the tea with honey will bolster its effect (no sweetening for diabetics).

Application: As required, drink one cup of tea 30 minutes to one hour before going to bed, for relief of tension. If used in a course of treatment, drink two to three cups of tea daily for four to eight weeks. For insomnia, drink one to two cups of tea in sips, unhurriedly, 30 minutes to one hour before bedtime.

● **Herbal baths**
Make the time for an herbal bath in the early evening, particularly if the evening "still has something in the offing." There are herbs (or ready-made bath additives) with natural essential oils that release tension, but at the same time act as a tonic (strengthen) and give vitality. These include lemon balm and lavender.

For an herbal bath that merely calms and relaxes, I recommend valerian; it also acts to produce sleep.

Because the preparation is simpler, I recommend that as a rule you use ready-made bath additives (available in health food stores and pharmacies), but you can, of course, also prepare your herbal bath yourself (see page 14).

Sleep Disturbances

In our hectic times, many people suffer from sleep disturbances: Some have trouble going to sleep, whereas others wake up after a short sleep and in despair get up and pace the floor in their home.

"I didn't sleep a wink all night, and I'm bushed" is a sentence we hear repeatedly. The feeling of being bushed is what causes the greatest suffering to people who have sleep disorders. A physical examination rarely leads to the discovery of a serious illness that results in sleeplessness.

Sleeping pills bring no lasting relief, but lead to dependency, stupefaction, and inactivity. A sleeping pill can even bring about the opposite of the result that its name promises. By lowering blood pressure and reducing the flow of blood to the brain, these pills can even unleash aggressions and anxieties.

Help from Medicinal Plants

Help is available, of course, in the form of medicinal plant applications. Because every person reacts differently, I would like to present several possibilities for you to try out. In this way you can find the application that helps you the most.

Problems Falling Asleep and Staying Asleep

● **Herbal pillow**
Often the herbal pillow alone will do the trick. It was in common use in earlier times, but then, with a condescending smile, it was dismissed as humbug—until recent studies rehabilitated the notion of herbal pillow therapy. Several medicinal plants have proved helpful as stuffing for such a pillow. The sequence in which I list them corresponds to my estimate of their worth: hop cones, St. John's wort (aerial parts), lavender flowers, lemon balm leaves, orange flowers, chamomile flowers, valerian roots, yarrow (aerial parts). Apart from the lavender, which often is

the sole component of a sleeping pillow, I consider blends of herbs more suitable. Try the following mixtures:

Herb Mix 1

Hop cone	1.05 (30)
Lavender flowers	.70 (20)
St. John's wort, aerial parts	.70 (20)

Herb Mix 2

Hop cones	.70 (20)
Valerian roots	.70 (20)
Yarrow, aerial parts	.35 (10)
Chamomile flowers	.35 (10)
Lemon balm leaves	.35 (10)

Herb Mix 3

Lemon balm leaves	.70 (20)
St. John's wort, aerial parts	.70 (20)
Valerian roots	.70 (20)
Lavender flowers	1.41 (40)

Herb Mix 4

Hop cones	1.41 (40)
Lavender flowers	1.41 (40)

Herb Mix 5

Hop cones	1.05 (30)
St. John's wort, aerial parts	1.05 (30)
Valerian roots	1.05 (30)

In general, one of these mixtures used as a pillow stuffing will retain its effect for one month.

How to prepare the little bag of herbs (herbal pillow) yourself: Using fine linen, sew a little square sack with sides that measure 4 inches (10 cm) to 6 inches (15 cm) in length. Provide one side with a zipper. Fill the sack loosely with the mix of your choosing, using enough herbs to make your pillow plump (don't fill it to bursting!). Put the herbal pillow either under your regular pillow or under the covers. You also can lay your head directly on it (but then you should put it in a pillow case).

The warmth of the bed will cause volatile substances to rise, and they will be inhaled, thus making their way into your body. With hops it is the 2-methyl-3-butene diol constituent that has a calming effect, even in small quantities. With other plants it is the essential oils that act as sedatives.

● **Sleeping-inducing drink**

A sleep-inducing drink also can help you, such as these two recipes:

Preparation 1: Bring 8 ounces (1/4 L) of whole milk mixed with 2 teaspoonfuls of crushed fennel seeds briefly to a boil. Strain to remove the milk "skin," and sweeten with 1 teaspoonful of honey (diabetics should not sweeten).

Preparation 2: Mix 8 ounces (1/4 L) of warm whole milk with an equal amount of warm chamomile tea (*Preparation,* see page 14), then add 1 to 2 teaspoonfuls of honey (diabetics should not sweeten).

Application: Drink one small cup of tea one hour before going to bed and another 30 minutes before bedtime; put the rest of your sleeping draft in a thermos bottle on your nightstand, to be drunk if you wake up during the night.

You also can use these recipes to prepare a sleep-inducing drink for your child (with children over age twelve, usually one half the adult dose is sufficient), to help him or her get ready to sleep if restless (see School Problems, Examination Phobia, Restlessness, page 97).

As an additional means to promote sleep— derived from an old book of home remedies—I would like to mention a sleeping draft that is somewhat tedious to make, to be sure, but has quite an impressive effect. At any rate, it is the equal of the valerian wine sold in pharmacies and health food stores in Europe as a remedy for insomnia. The instructions for *preparation and application* appear as they did in the book of home remedies:

"Very carefully weigh out .35 ounces (10 g) of valerian roots, .35 ounces (10 g) of hop cones, .35 ounces (10 g) of lemon balm leaves, .35 ounces (10 g) of St. John's wort, and .35 ounces (10 g) of lavender flowers. Pulverize everything as well as possible in a mortar. Then pour the mixture into a large bottle, and pour 1 quart (1 L) of red wine over the pulverized medicinal herbs. Put this initial mixture aside for ten days, remembering to shake the bottle once a day. After five days add a small stick of cinnamon. Once a total of ten days has passed, strain the mixture through a piece of clean flannel (a coffee filter can be substituted) and pour it into another bottle. This sleeping potion will keep for several weeks. When unable to sleep, drink one small glass (about 50 to 100 milliliters) of it 30 minutes before going to bed. This will help you fall asleep, and your wait for sleep to come will no longer be tormenting and filled with melancholy thoughts, but will seem pleasantly relaxing."

● **Valerian tea**
Valerian tea (*Preparation*, see page 14) also is a time-tested sleep inducer. Nondiabetics can sweeten it with honey. If you prefer valerian drops (available in some pharmacies and health food stores): Add the dose recommended on the label to a glass of warm water. Take this sleeping draft 30 minutes before going to bed.

Although the last two suggestions are intended chiefly for adults, valerian tea also is applicable to children, for whom it can be equally helpful (see School Problems, Examination Phobia, Restlessness, page 97). Valerian wine is not recommended for children.

● **Valerian bath**
A valerian bath is also an excellent means of promoting sleep (*Preparation*, see page 25).

Feeling of Oppression

● **Tea blend**
If you can't sleep because your heart is drawing attention to itself through nervous disorders (irregular heartbeat, feeling of oppression or constriction in the heart area), or if you are troubled by anxieties at night, then I recommend this tea for you:

Hawthorn flowers	1.05 (30)
Lemon balm leaves	.70 (20)
St. John's wort, aerial parts	.70 (20)
Valerian roots	.35 (10)

Preparation, see page 14.

Application: In the morning and at noon, drink one cup of unsweetened tea; 30 minutes before going to bed in the evening drink one cup of tea sweetened with 1 to 2 teaspoonfuls of honey (not applicable to diabetics!). Sip the tea slowly.

The hawthorn flowers in this tea assist the action of the other calmative medicinal plants by strengthening the agitated heart and eliminating the irregularity of its beat. This in turn diminishes the feelings of anxiety.

St. John's wort is considered effective for mild depressions and states of anxiety.

Additional Recommendations

● **Coffee or glucose**
As absurd as it may sound: If your sleep disturbance is attributable to overly low blood pressure and thus to a reduced flow of blood to the brain, a cup of coffee—sweetened with honey and drunk just before bedtime—will help! (This remedy is not suitable for diabetics!) You really should try this simple application. Coffee improves the cerebral blood supply, and honey provides plenty of glucose. Glucose deficiency in the brain can be a cause of sleep disturbances.

Older people, for example, who wake up at night and for hours are unable to go back to sleep, also find it helpful to eat a piece of chocolate or—even better—a piece of hard (sugar) candy; sleep will not be long in coming (not suitable for diabetics!).

● **Appreciate beauty**
Try to let your troubles go, and make a conscious effort to notice and enjoy all the forms of beauty that we encounter repeatedly each day. Many of the worries that vex us during the night—when looked at in the daytime, when you are rested and relaxed—are not so great as they may seem in the dark of night. Older people in particular often feel alone; because they don't do much and often isolate themselves, they lack someone who will respond to them and to whom

they can unburden themselves. All of us, however, need friends who can provide a boost.

Everyone—that is, everyone who wants to—also can look for some truly useful activity; then we feel needed, rather than "put on the shelf." If we do something that brings pleasure to ourselves and others, we feel tired after a job well done and are able to sleep soundly. This "job" may be a hobby that we pursue, either with others who share our interests or alone; it may be a walk or a hike. A dog for whose care we are responsible, a dog that forces us to "take it outdoors," may provide a remedy for people who have trouble sleeping. There are any number of possibilities! It always is just a matter of finding the right one.

● **Cold sponge bath**
Another effective way of promoting sleep is the cold sponge bath treatment. It is quite simple: With a cloth that has been dipped into room-temperature water and squeezed out, sponge off your entire body, but do not dry it. Then go immediately to bed and cover yourself up well.

Neurodystonia

Often we also use the older term neurasthenia (nervous debility and exhaustion) for a complex of symptoms with great range and diversity.

Symptoms and Their Causes

The most common symptoms of neurodystonia are palpitations, oppression of the heart, states of restlessness and anxiety, sleeplessness, dizziness, headaches, and damp, clammy hands and feet. Many patients manifest all these symptoms, others, only a few. The severity of the symptoms varies greatly; the problems also intensify when the patient feels hurt or offended or when something unexpected is in store. Therefore we can say that anyone who has neurodystonia suffers equally from physical and mental stress and strain.

What is neurodystonia? It is not a disease per se—what we feel are reactions at various sites in our body; their causes must be sought in an imbalance of the autonomic nervous system.

The autonomic nervous system is the totality of the nerve cells (neurons) and ganglion cells (gangliocytes). It regulates the vital functions; it ensures that respiration, digestion, glandular secretion, and water balance are "right." We cannot influence our autonomic nervous system through our will (except in persons trained in biofeedback teachings or meditation), and only the symptoms listed tell us that it is not in equilibrium. A physician, even after a thorough examination, will find no organic disease. Nevertheless, the patient really does feel sick, and this feeling often focuses on a particular organ (stomach, heart) or on the extremities.

Whether neurodystonia is inborn or acquired through particular experiences or ways of living (stress) has not yet been determined.

Help from Medicinal Plants

Medicinal herbs can be used to treat these troublesome and "alarming" symptoms as well! It is possible to lessen overreactions of the autonomic nervous system without using strong agents. Sometimes it is advisable to give particular attention to whatever organ is displaying the most severe reactions (heart, stomach). Usually, however, it is preferable to "suppress" the entire overreactive autonomic nervous system.

Please note

If you sense irritation in the heart or stomach area, you should never try to medicate yourself until your doctor has determined beyond all doubt that no organic damage is present In any event, inform your physician of your intention to treat yourself with natural medicines.

Because the perception of the trouble and the feeling of illness associated with it vary from one person to another, you will have to experiment a bit to find the recipe that is right for you.

Palpitations

● **Valerian**
If it is your heart that is causing you the most trouble by palpitating or beating irregularly, valerian drops (available in pharmacies; follow directions on the label), can bring marked relief promptly.
Preparation, see page 14.
Application: Drink three cups of tea per day.

● **Tea blend**
is tea also has proved reliable:

Valerian roots	1.05 (30)
Hawthorn flowers	.70 (20)
Lemon balm leaves	.35 (10)

Preparation, see page 14.
Application: Drink one cup of tea three times a day.

Stomach Trouble

● **Lemon balm tea**
If it is your stomach ("everything upsets my stomach") that is having a nervous reaction, then I think lemon balm tea is especially suitable. It will calm, relax spasms, settle your stomach, and promote digestion.
Preparation: Pour 8 ounces (1/4 L) of boiling water over three heaping teaspoonfuls of lemon balm leaves, let steep, covered, for ten minutes, then strain.
Application: Drink three cups of tea between meals. If you drink a fourth cup before bedtime, you will go to sleep easily. Instead of lemon balm tea, you also may drink chamomile tea (*Preparation and application*, see page 14).

Lack of Appetite

● **Tea blend**
If you suffer from lack of appetite also, then I recommend this tea:

Chamomile flowers	.70 (20)
Lemon balm leaves	.70 (20)
Peppermint leaves	.17 (5)
Hop cones	.17 (5)
European centaury, aerial parts	.17 (5)

Preparation, see page 14.
Application: Drink one small cup of tea 30 minutes before each meal.

Insomnia and Anxiety

● **Tea blend**
If sleeplessness and a state of anxiety predominate, then I recommend this tea:

St. John's wort, aerial parts	1.05 (30)
Lemon balm leaves	.70 (20)
Hop cones	.35 (10)
Lavender flowers	.17 (5)
Orange flowers	.17 (5)

Preparation, see page 14.

Application: Three times a day, slowly sip one cup of very warm tea. A course of treatment should last at least four weeks.

Herbal Baths for Relaxation

To calm the disturbed autonomic nervous system and to allay the numerous complaints, medicinal baths are especially helpful. In my opinion, a lavender bath or a lavender-oil bath, available in pharmacies, ranks in first place.

A hayseed bath (*Preparation,* see below) is also suitable—I recommend it particularly to women experiencing menopause (see page 107).

You also can use the lavender bath and the hayseed bath in alternation.

The bath therapy can by supported with a course of treatment with tea. There are many herbs that are appropriate: lemon balm, valerian, St. John's wort, passionflower plants, or hop cones.

Two or three times a week, take a bath—followed by at least two hours of bed rest.

Preparation and application of the recommended tension easing baths—the amounts given are sufficient for one bath:

● **Valerian bath**
Pour 2 quarts (2 L) of water over 3.52 ounces (100 g) of valerian roots (valerian tea), bring to a boil, let boil for ten minutes, then strain. Add the extract to the bath water. You also can add 3.52 ounces (100 mL) of tincture of valerian (obtainable from pharmacies and health food stores) to the bath water. Temperature of bath water, 95 to 100.4°F (35–38°C); length of bath, 10 to 15 minutes. Rest after bathing.

● **Oat straw bath**
Pour 3 to 5 quarts (3–5 L) of water over 3.52 to 5.29 ounces (100–150 g) of cut up (chopped) oat straw, bring to a boil, let boil for about 20 minutes, then strain. Add the extract to the bath water.

Temperature of bath water, 95 to 100.4°F (35–38°C); length of bath, 10 to 15 minutes. Rest after bathing.

● **Hayseed bath**
Pour 5 quarts (5 L) of water over 10.58 to 17.63 ounces (300–500 g) of hayseed, bring to a boil, let boil for about 15 minutes, then strain. Add the extract to the bath water.

Temperature of bath water, 95 to 100.4°F (35–37°C); length of bath, 10 to 15 minutes. Rest after bathing.

● **Hops bath**
Pour 3 quarts (3 L) of water over 1.76 ounces (50 g) of hop cones, bring to a boil, let steep for about 20 minutes, then strain. Add the extract to the bath water.

Temperature of bath water, 95 to 100.4°F (35–38°C); length of bath, 10 to 15 minutes. Rest after bathing.

● **Lavender bath**
Pour 1 quart (1 L) of boiling water over 1.76 to 2.11 ounces (50–60 g) of lavender flowers, let steep for 20 minutes, then strain. Add the extract to the bath water.

Temperature of bath water, 95 to 100.4°F (35–38°C); length of bath, 10 to 15 minutes. Rest after bathing.

● **Lemon balm bath**
Pour 5 quarts (5 L) of boiling water over 2.11 to 2.46 ounces (60–70 g) of lemon balm leaves, let steep for about 20 minutes, then strain. Add the extract to the bath water.

Temperature of bath water, 95 to 100.4°F (35–38°C); length of bath, 10 to 15 minutes. Rest after bathing.

You also can buy ready-made bath additives (available in pharmacies). It is important, however, to distinguish between cosmetic baths and medicinal baths; you need to make sure that the essential oils from the herbs are present in sufficient amounts in the bath additive.

As an Alterative (substance that speeds healing)

● **Tea blend**

The following tea elicits such high praise from everyone who tastes it that I want to recommend it especially:

Hawthorn flowers	.35 (10)
St. John's wort, aerial parts	1.05 (30)
Lemon balm leaves	1.05 (30)
Hop cones	.35 (10)
Orange flowers	.35 (10)
Lavender flowers	.35 (10)
Hibiscus flowers	.35 (10)

Preparation: Pour 8 ounces (1/4 L) of boiling water over 2 heaping teaspoonfuls of the blend, let steep in a covered container for five minutes, then strain.

Application: Both morning and noon, after eating, sip one cup of tea, as warm as possible.

In the evening use 3 heaping teaspoonfuls (instead of 2) to prepare the tea, and sweeten it with honey (diabetics don't sweeten). Sip the tea, as warm as possible, 30 minutes before bedtime, in an atmosphere of tranquility.

After a course of treatment lasting four to eight weeks, a favorable change usually has been brought about—a toning down of the autonomic nervous system, whereby the symptoms diminish noticeably or possibly vanish altogether. Many people have told me that optimism and zest for living reappeared after such a treatment.

The tea treatment may be repeated after an interval of two to four weeks.

Please note

During storage the hop cones will shed their glands, which are concealed by scales. The glands, in the form of a fine yellow powder, will be deposited on the bottom of the storage container. These glands play an essential role in the effectiveness of hop. To ensure that all the servings of tea are of equal strength, I recommend that you first grind (mortar and pestle) the cones to a "tea cut" before storing them. Then give the container in which the drug is stored a thorough shake (to distribute it equally) each time you remove some hops.

Because of the high proportion of St. John's wort in this blend, do not sunbathe or undergo ultraviolet or solarium therapy during the treatment; St. John's wort increases the skin's sensitivity to sunlight.

● **Mixture of drops**

If you do not want to try the suggested course of treatment with tea—for example, because you believe you lack the time—you can also try drops. Your pharmacist or health food store can obtain these for you and you can mix them yourself in the following proportions:

Avena (oatmeal) homeopathic drops (1x)	1.05 (30)
Passiflora (passionflower) homeopathic drops (1x)	1.05 (30)
Tincture of bitter orange (*Tinctura Aurantii*)	.35 (10)
Tincture of valerian (*Tinctura Valerianae*)	.35 (10)

Application: Twice a day, put 10 to 20 drops on sugar (diabetics put drops in water) and swallow; at bedtime it is advisable to double these amounts.

Season It Well

An additional piece of advice relating to neurodystonia will surely come as a great surprise to you. I claim that liberal use of seasonings—particularly spicy and bitter, aromatic seasonings—relieves suffering.

I recommend that you use paprika (up to level 5 on the Hungarian scale, the kind sold as "rose paprika"), pepper, ginger, galangal, turmeric, cinnamon, cloves, nutmeg, mustard (including hot mustard), mugwort, marjoram, thyme, basil, lemon balm, peppermint, and peel of bitter oranges.

Use of hearty seasonings will not place a burden on the stomach, despite previous assumptions, nor will it stimulate abnormal production of acids in the stomach or damage the kidneys.

On the contrary, generous use of seasonings will lessen the strain on the circulatory system, increase cardiac activity, and promote the fermentation of almost all the gastric juices. If you want a higher level of vitality and a more intense experience of life, I recommend that you use plenty of hearty seasonings—particularly if you suffer from nervous exhaustion. Experiment with all the many spices and herbs that we have available—for the good of your health!

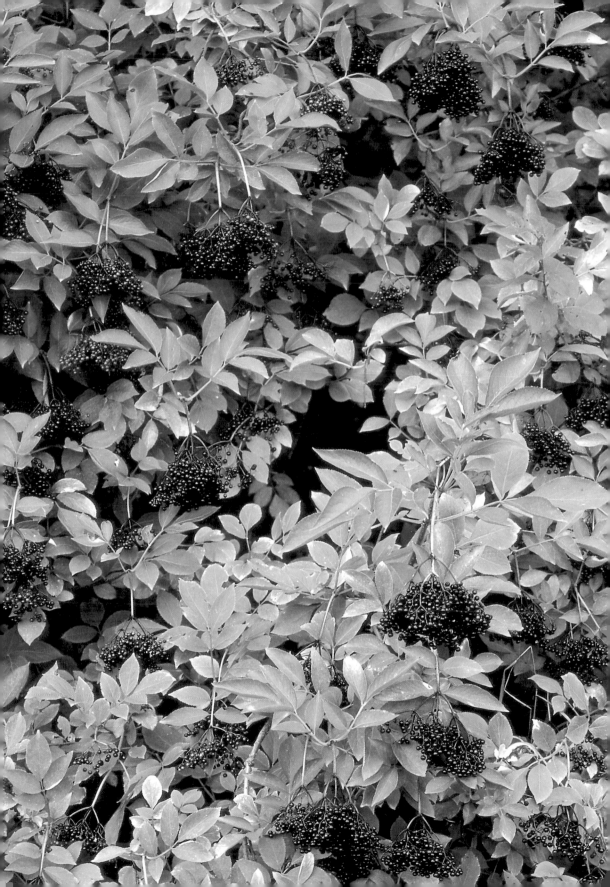

Colds

← *Elderberry*

An Ounce of Prevention Is Worth a Pound of Cure

Few diseases and health disturbances can be prevented as successfully as the cold, or "flu," as laymen say. (This usage refers to flulike infections, not true viral influenza.) Almost everyone gets a cold once or twice a year. We have become so accustomed to having a head cold, a scratchy throat, and/or a cough during the winter months that we consider these infections inevitable and harmless and take no special pains to prevent them. When a change is heard in the voice of a coworker, a neighbor sneezes or coughs, and many children are absent from kindergarten or from school, the "flu" is going around, and it is only a matter of time "until we catch it too."

Strengthening Resistance

I maintain that it doesn't have to happen! If we strengthen our body's powers of resistance, it will be hard for the pathogens (most of which are viruses) to get a foothold.

We build up our resistance through hardening our bodies—for example, by taking a walk in all kinds of weather or by making sure that our home and office are not overheated and are ventilated frequently. Nutrition also is important in warding off infections: Vegetables, salads, and plenty of fresh fruit should dominate our menus. Regular visits to a sauna also build up resistance. If we can also keep from shaking hands with infected people and avoid using a shared towel after washing our hands, we can escape contagion in most cases.

In addition, by getting plenty of sleep and avoiding all unusual exertion, we help our immune system fend off infectious diseases. It is important, too, to dress appropriately and make sure that our feet stay warm and dry. Then if we also promote a stimulating, stabilizing herbal tea to the status of "house tea," we will be well protected and able to face the damp, cold winter weather with an easy mind.

Help from Healing Plants

The number of medicinal plants that are effective in treating colds is so vast that I had to make a selection. In the following material I recommend only those medicinal plants with which I have over 40 years of experience, plants that are tolerated well. In most cases they also are acknowledged as efficacious by scientists. You will encounter some of them elsewhere, too, as many medicinal plants are employed against several, often quite diverse, complaints. Thyme, for example, is a traditional stomachic, but it is just as useful in relieving dry cough and whooping cough.

The medicinal plants recommended here are sufficient to deal with all cold symptoms.

Elderberry flowers, English plantain, European cowslip roots, fennel seeds, Iceland moss, linden flowers, marshmallow roots, mullein, sage leaves, and the aerial parts of thyme—in alphabetical order—are my favorites. To support their effect I also like to use rose hips, with their high vitamin content, lemon balm leaves, and chamomile flowers.

You may wonder why coltsfoot is not on my list. In fact, coltsfoot leaf tea is an excellent cough remedy, but it contains minute, variable amounts of pyrrolizidine alkaloids. In higher concentrations, these alkaloids can damage the liver, and they are also said to be carcinogenic.

Thus far there is no clear proof that people have suffered any harm from drinking coltsfoot tea as a cold or cough remedy, but for the sake of caution I have replaced coltsfoot in all my recipes with Iceland moss and high mallow flowers or high mallow leaves, which, like coltsfoot, contain plentiful amounts of soothing plant mucilage. Iceland moss, moreover, has a tonic and antibacterial effect due to the bitter lichenic acids it contains. On page 179 I present a detailed description of this reliable medicinal plant, which was long forgotten.

For Prevention

● **Tea blends**

Here are three recipes for tea blends that you can use to ward off colds. The teas are quite delicious, and may be used as a mealtime beverage.

Tea Blend 1	oz. (g)
Elderberry flower	.70 (20)
Rose hips (without seeds)	70 (20)
Lemon balm leaves	.70 (20)
Raspberry leaves	1.41 (40)

Tea Blend 2	
Linden flowers	88 (25)
Lemon balm leaves	.88 (25)
Chamomile flowers	.70 (20)
Hibiscus flowers	.70 (20)

Tea Blend 3	
Iceland moss	.70 (20)
Chamomile flowers	.35 (10)
Blackberry leaves	.70 (20)
Rose hips (with seeds)	1.76 (50)

Preparation of these tea blends: Pour 1 quart (1 L) of boiling water over 3 heaping teaspoonfuls of whichever blend you choose, let steep for five minutes, then strain.

Application: Drink three to five cups of tea per day. It is even more effective if sweetened with honey (diabetics do not sweeten).

At the First Signs of Discomfort

As a rule, flulike infections (colds) begin slowly. We notice "that something is not quite right." The mucous membranes that line the mouth and throat are dry, and a scratchy or slightly burning sensation is felt in the throat. Alternatively, the mucous membranes of the nose are dry, we have to sneeze, there is a tickling sensation when we breathe through our nose, and the mucous membranes at the back of the nose, on the uvula, and in the throat feel sore. If you react without delay, you generally can ward off a flulike infection now.

● **Progressively hot footbath**

A footbath is first on the list. Follow the procedures described on page 14.

● **Sudorific teas**

To bolster your resistance, I recommend that the footbath be followed by a linden flower tea or an elderberry flower tea (*Preparation*, see page 74). Both teas are considered sudorifics, but if you drink them only moderately warm and in sips, profuse perspiration will not result.

● **Tea blend**

The following tea blend also has proved useful for these purposes:

Lemon balm leaves	70 (20)
Elderberry flowers	.70 (20)
Iceland moss	.35 (10)
Rose hips	1.05 (30)

Preparation and application, see page 14. Sweetening with honey is recommended (diabetics do not sweeten).

● **Teas for gargling**

You can "counter" the incipient infection even more thoroughly by gargling with sage tea, thyme tea, and chamomile tea (*Preparation*, see page 14) in rotation. If you gargle three times a day, each tea will be used once; the sequence is unimportant.

Every medicinal plant has an effect peculiar to it, an effect that sets it apart from other plants. In the right combination, therefore, medicinal plants can be helpful for a great number of different complaints that may appear at the start of a cold.

● **Thyme bath**

A thyme bath (see page 39) before bedtime also helps the body ward off the first signs of infection.

Cold Symptoms and Their Treatment

If you started the preventive measures too late and failed to fend off the infection, then you need to alleviate the troublesome symptoms. Medicinal plant applications are well suited for this purpose.

Important: It is essential to keep in mind the limits of self-medication (see page 7). Stronger means sometimes are called for, and your physician will specify these. Supportive therapy with medicinal plants, however, is always appropriate.

Sore Throat

A scratchy throat, difficulty in swallowing, and inflamed mucous membranes in the throat are especially unpleasant.

● Marshmallow tea
With marshmallow tea, which contains a great deal of plant mucilage, you can soothe the pain quickly. The marshmallow mucilage forms a protective coating on the inflamed mucosae of the mouth and throat. Swallowing becomes much less problematic. Under the protective layer of plant mucilage, the inflammation has a chance to heal undisturbed.

Marshmallow tea has to be prepared with cold water, because the plant's root contains a large amount of starch along with the desirable mucilage. Because of the starch content, pouring boiling water on the roots would cause the cells to stick together, and the sought-after mucilage would not find its way into the tea.

Preparation: Pour 8 ounces (1/4 L) of cold water over 1 tablespoonful of chopped marshmallow roots and let steep for two to three hours, stirring occasionally. After being strained, the tea can be heated to drinking temperature.

Application: It is best to sip two to three cups of marshmallow tea slowly each day; this way the soothing marshmallow mucilage will be able to reach even the farthest corners of the mouth. In addition, you can use the tea as a gargle and a mouthwash.

● Iceland moss tea
Iceland moss, with its high mucilage content, has a similar effect. It too can be used to prepare a tea for drinking or gargling. There are two ways to prepare the infusion properly:

Preparation 1: Pour 8 ounces (1/4 L) of boiling water over 2 teaspoonfuls of the chopped drug, let steep for ten minutes, then strain.

Preparation 2: Pour 8 ounces (1/4 L) of boiling water over 2 teaspoonfuls of the chopped drug and strain after 30 seconds. Discard the liquid, which contains bitter constituents almost exclusively. Once again pour 8 ounces (1/4 L) of boiling water over the drug, let steep for 10 to 15 seconds, then strain.

The second infusion contains fewer bitter constituents and is therefore better suited for children. In this method of preparation, however, the antibiotic effect of the lichenic acids is largely lost; adults, at least, should choose the first method of preparing the tea.

● Helpful recommendations
Once an infection is under way, it is also advisable to gargle with sage tea, thyme tea, and chamomile tea in rotation, to disinfect the mouth and throat area.

Hoarseness

With hoarseness, the vocal cords are affected. For this reason, try to talk as little as possible if you are hoarse. Warm throat compresses and warm drinks—as warm as you can bear—are the best initial therapy.

● Hot teas
With hot drinks it is not the quantity of liquid that matters; the important thing is to drink something hot with great frequency (every 30 minutes, if possible). It is best to drink chamomile tea and Iceland moss tea in

alternation, because they complement each other in their effect.

Preparation, see page 14.

● **Throat compress**

A throat compress is an especially good remedy for hoarseness. According to an old recipe for this household remedy, the compress should be prepared from potatoes. Experience has proved it superior to the simple hot water compress because it retains heat better.

Preparation and application: Boil three to five potatoes until they are soft and mash them while they are still warm. Wrap the mashed potatoes in a thin piece of cloth and place the compress around your neck so that it reaches from the chin to the shoulders. Wrap a woolen cloth around it. Leave it in place until it has lost its warmth. You can apply such a compress three to five times a day without misgivings. Be careful with the temperature of the potatoes! They should be no hotter than you can easily tolerate if they are placed on the inside of your arm. Try it out in advance!

● **Chamomile tea inhalant**

An additional therapy is the inhalation of steam from chamomile tea (*Preparation,* see page 14) or from water containing 1/4 teaspoonful of Epsom Salts. (*Application,* see page 14).

Please note

In cases of high fever (above 102.2°F [39°C]) and persistent throat pain, or if the tonsils are badly swollen, consult a physician.

Head Cold

A nasal catarrh, or cold in the head, probably is the most frequent symptom of the common cold. Once a head cold has become entrenched, it is difficult to get rid of. If untreated, a head cold will last seven days, and if treated, one week, as an old folk saying tells us. In old books of household remedies we often read: "Head colds are three days in coming, three days in staying, and three days in going."

We are not quite so helpless in dealing with the nasal catarrh as it would appear, however. We can ease the symptoms, open the stuffy nose, improve the runny nose, and shorten the duration of the discomfort. A true cure, however, is offered neither by classical medicine nor by naturopathy; the viruses that cause colds in the head are largely resistant to natural remedies.

● **Tea blend**

When a head cold is just getting started, promptly drink a tea for colds and take a footbath in progressively hot water (see page 14). In the evening, a chamomile tea or thyme tea inhalation is highly recommended.

Rose hips (with seeds)	.70 (20)
Elderberry flowers	.49 (14)
Chamomile flowers	.49 (14)
Linden flowers	.49 (14)
Blackberry leaves	.38 (11)
Sage leaves	35 (10)
Willow bark	.35 (10)
Hibiscus flowers	.17 (5)

Preparation: Pour 8 ounces (1/4 L) of boiling water over 3 teaspoonfuls of this blend and let steep for five minutes. Sweetening with honey is recommended (except for diabetics).

● **Homeopathic remedies**

Also recommended are two traditional homeopathic remedies for head colds, both made from medicinal plants: *Nux vomica,* for a stuffy nose and scratchy throat; *Allium cepa,* a homeopathic medicine made from the common onion, for a "runny nose" with a dripping secretion that causes sores.

Application: Three to six times each day, take 5 to 10 drops of the sixth decimal potency (6x) of *Allium cepa* in some water; alternatively, five to ten pellets (alcohol-free). Infants should be given one pellet of the fourth decimal potency (4x) every two hours; older children get 2 drops 4x every hour.

Frontal and Paranasal Sinusitis

If you leave the head cold untreated, the pathogens may make their way into the sinuses and establish themselves there. A dull sensation of pressure in the area of the paranasal sinuses or a headache in the forehead area are the first signs of such a development. Secondary infections of this kind are quite stubborn.

Please note

I strongly advise you to consult your physician at once if you notice these symptoms.

● **Inhalations with teas or essential oils**

You can assist your doctor's therapy through frequent inhalations using chamomile tea, thyme tea (*Preparation,* see page 14), or the following essential oils, which you can mix once the ingredients are obtained:

Dwarf-pine oil	.17 (5)
Eucalyptus oil	.10 (3)
Thyme oil	.07 (2)

Preparation: Add 3 to 5 drops to the water for the inhalant (*Application*, see page 14).

● **Teas for colds**

Drinking large quantities of the tea for colds listed under Head Cold (see page 33) also will help ease the discomfort.

● **Honeycombs**

Folk medicine recommends that one chew a small piece of real honeycomb that still contains plenty of honey. Honeycomb is available in health food stores (not suitable for diabetics).

Coughs

Not all coughs are alike. If you want to successfully treat your cough with teas made from medicinal plants, you need to be able to tell a dry cough from a cough with viscid bronchial mucus. A cough that is an attendant symptom of a cold will respond nicely to self-treatment with medicinal teas. After only a few cups of tea you will feel some relief, and soon the cough will be gone. Left untreated, it often can hang on for weeks.

A cough is not always an attendant symptom of a common cold, however; serious bronchial and pulmonary problems also result in a cough. In such cases, of course, treatment by a physician is imperative.

Please note

If you suffer from a cough and have a high fever (over 102.2°F [39°C]) at the same time, see your physician at once. Medical intervention is also necessary if the cough is not gone after one week, despite your treatment, or if it returns once the tea therapy is discontinued.

Dry Cough

If, when going from indoors to outdoors, from a warm room to a cold one, or vice versa, you are suddenly plagued with fairly prolonged fits of coughing that bring tears to your eyes, or if you get such a paroxysm of coughing without fore-warning when you speak, then you have a dry cough. A cough of this kind results when the mucous membranes of the throat or bronchial tubes are involved. Medicinal plants with a high mucilage content will bring relief.

● **Marshmallow tea, Iceland moss tea**
Marshmallow tea (*Preparation,* see page 32) is a good remedy: Several times a day, drink a cup of freshly made, warmed marshmallow tea.

Iceland moss tea (*Preparation,* see page 32) has a similar effect. Drink a cup of it several times daily.

Whether these teas should be sweetened with honey or not is debatable. I consider honey so important for anyone with a cold accompanied by a cough that I advise its use as a sweetener (except for diabetics, of course). Others, however, are of the opinion that honey irritates the injured mucous membranes in the mouth and throat. Try honey and see how you react.

● **Tea blend**
A tea blend for dry coughs has the following ingredients:

English plantain leaves	.70 (20)
High mallow flowers	.70 (20)
Lemon balm leaves	.70 (20)
Raspberry leaves	.70 (20)

Preparation, see page 14.
Application: Drink three to five cups of tea daily, as needed.

Spasmodic Cough, Whooping Cough

Spasmodic coughs, or whooping coughs in children, are characterized by fits of coughing in which the muscles used for respiration contract spasmodically, resulting in great difficulty in breathing.

● **Thyme tea**
In both cases, a tea made from thyme has consistently had a soothing effect. The essential oils in the thyme are able to reduce convulsibility considerably. In addition, thyme acts as a disinfectant in the areas of the upper respiratory passages and the lungs, an effect due to the thymol in thyme oil.

Preparation, see page 14.
Application: Three to five times a day, drink one cup of tea with or without honey (for diabetics, without honey).

In addition, use thyme tea as an inhalant (see page 34) and take a thyme bath (see page 39) two or three times a week.

● **Tea blend**
The following blend has proved helpful for adults with fits of spasmodic coughing.

Thyme, aerial parts	1.05 (30)
English plantain leaves	1.05 (30)
Chamomile flowers	.70 (20)
European cowslip roots	.35 (10)
(for people over age sixty)	(.70 [20])

Preparation, see page 14.
Application: Drink five to six cups of tea, as warm as possible, each day.

Cough with Viscid Mucus

You hear a rattle when you inhale and exhale, and there is a tickle in your throat that makes you cough; despite violent coughing, however, you are unable to bring up any phlegm. Bronchial tubes that are thus congested with mucus are an ideal breeding ground for germs. Therefore it is extremely important to loosen the viscid mucus so that it can be coughed up.

Some medicinal plants that contain saponins are good for that purpose, because these substances reduce the surface tension of the mucus, which is loosened as a result. In addition, the saponins stimulate the gastric mucosa, which—via the vagus nerve—causes in the bronchial tubes a secretion that "lifts" the viscid mucus coating. Improved ability to expectorate the phlegm is brought about by other medicinal plants (fennel, for example).

● **Tea blends**
In the treatment of such coughs, tea blends are superior to teas brewed from single medicinal plants, because it is important to trigger several operative mechanisms simultaneously. There are many effective blends. Here are three recipes I consider best. Try them all, and stick with the blend that you think works (and tastes) best.

Tea Blend 1

European cowslip roots	1.05 (30)
English plantain leaves	1.05 (30)
Fennel seeds (crushed)	1.05 (30)
Iceland moss	.70 (20)
Elderberry flowers	.70 (20)
Rose hips (with seeds)	.70 (20)
High mallow flowers	.35 (10)

Tea Blend 2

Mullein flowers	1.05 (30)
Linden flowers	.70 (20)
English plantain leaves	.70 (20)
Fennel seeds (crushed)	.70 (20)
European cowslip roots	.35 (10)
High mallow leaves	.35 (10)

Tea Blend 3

European cowslip roots	.70 (20)
Linden flowers	.70 (20)
Chamomile flowers	.70 (20)
Lemon balm leaves	.35 (10)

Preparation of these tea blends, see page 14.

Application: Drink four cups of tea during the course of the day, and drink one more just before bedtime.

Hybrid Forms of Coughs

A cough that accompanies a cold is not always clearly identifiable as one of the types discussed thus far. Often the sufferers have both a dry cough and excessive congestion.

● **Tea blends**

For such cases I recommend tea blends with a broad effect. Here are four such mixtures:

Tea Blend 1
This blend is recommended if it is the congestion that is causing you the most discomfort:

English plantain leaves	1.05 (30)
European cowslip roots	.70 (20)
Linden flowers	.70 (20)
Lemon balm leaves	.35 (10)
Thyme, aerial parts	.35 (10)
Chamomile flowers	.35 (10)
High mallow flowers	.35 (10)

Tea Blend 2
This blend is recommended if the tickling in your throat bothers you most:

Iceland moss	1.05 (30)
Mullein flowers or leaves	.70 (20)
English plantain leaves	.35 (10)
Elderberry flowers	.35 (10)
Thyme, aerial parts	.35 (10)
High mallow leaves	.35 (10)

Tea Blend 3
This blend should be tried by people whose discomfort is due in equal proportions to a dry cough and to congestion:

Fennel seeds (crushed)	1.05 (30)
Iceland moss	.70 (20)
Mullein flowers or leaves	.35 (10)
Linden flowers	.35 (10)
English plantain leaves	.35 (10)
Sage leaves	.35 (10)
Rose hips (with seeds)	.35 (10)

Preparation of these three tea blends, see page 14.
Application: Several times a day, drink one cup of tea, as warm as possible, sweetened with honey (no honey for diabetics).

Doctors recommend that we drink large amounts of hot liquids—up to 1.5 quarts (1.5 L) per day—for colds of all kinds, especially those accompanied by a cough and mild bronchitis. For this purpose I recommend the following tea:

Tea Blend 4

Raspberry leaves	.70 (20)
Blackberry leaves	.70 (20)
Lemon balm leaves	.70 (20)
Chamomile flowers	.70 (20)
Mullein flowers or leaves	.35 (10)
Iceland moss	.35 (10)
English plantain leaves	.35 (10)
Elderberry flowers	.17 (5)
Linden flowers	.17 (5)
Thyme, aerial parts	.17 (5)
Rose hips (with seeds)	1.23 (35)

Preparation, see page 14. You can prepare several cups of tea at a time to have in reserve, keeping the tea warm in a thermos bottle.

Application: Sip one small cup of very warm tea every hour. Because of the large amount to be consumed daily, please drink the tea unsweetened; otherwise, you would be getting too many carbohydrates (calories!).

Fever

Almost every cold is accompanied by a slight fever. This is the body's defense reaction—a natural and healing process. Do not try to reduce elevated temperatures unless they exceed 102.2°F (39°C) and last longer than three days.

> **Please note**
>
> If your fever climbs above 102.2°F (39°C) or lasts more than three days, call the doctor without delay!

● **With fever, drink plenty of liquids**

The prime necessity for anyone with a fever is to drink large quantities of liquids. In addition to the tea blend recommended (see page 33), these may include cool, refreshing fruit juices that are high in vitamins, but unsweetened. You need to drink a total of 1.5 to 2 quarts (1.5–2 L) of liquids daily.

To Build Up Resistance

● **Sweat cure**

At one time it was customary to begin the treatment of cold sufferers with a sweat cure, in order to nip the infection in the bud by strengthening the body's own powers of resistance. Today the value or lack of value of such a procedure is contested. Some argue that it is too arduous for patients to undergo and that the effect is not convincing. I disagree. It is true that a sweat cure places strain on the circulatory system—but the effect is beneficial.

> **Please note**
>
> If you suffer from circulatory instability, if your heart is weakened, or if you are over fifty years old, it is essential to ask your doctor whether a sweat cure is advisable for you!

Even if you have a stable circulatory system and a healthy heart, you must not undertake a sweat cure when alone! Because of the burden it places on your circulation, someone has to be present to help you if necessary.

Patients have to be observed closely while they sweat, so that the treatment can be interrupted immediately if circulatory problems become apparent. The first indications are blue lips or a pale face. A cup of coffee (with absolutely no alcohol added!) will quickly get the patient's circulation back in order. If that doesn't work, call a doctor at once. A sweat cure should not be performed on a daily basis. It is advisable to implement one at the onset of the illness and possibly also at its end, if the illness was lengthy.

How to implement a sweat cure: Prepare 1 pint (1/2 L) of sudorific tea from 2 heaping teaspoonfuls of linden flowers and an equal amount of elderberry flowers, over which you pour 1 pint (1/2 L) of boiling water. Let steep for ten minutes, then strain. Drink this tea as hot as you can bear it and as quickly as possible. Then take a bath (a hayseed bath is especially good—see page 39), initially in water at 98.6°F (37°C), which you quickly raise to 104°F (40°C) by adding hot water. Spend about three minutes in the 104°F (40°C) water. Then let the water drip off your body, wrap yourself in a large, heated bath towel, and lie down—well wrapped in a wool blanket—in your bed, with an additional blanket on top. After a short time you will begin to sweat. The sweat cure, which should last 30 minutes at most, begins at the moment the first beads of sweat appear on your forehead. After sweating, dry yourself thoroughly. Finally, rest at least one hour in fresh, prewarmed sheets.

Herbal Baths for Colds

Here are several herbal baths, some of which I have recommended in the applications in this chapter. They all will help ease your discomfort. Try them and see which bath helps you most.

How to prepare baths for colds—the amounts given are for one bath:

● **Eucalyptus bath**

Pour 3 quarts (3 L) of water over 2.11 to 2.46 ounces (60–70 g) of eucalyptus leaves, bring to a boil, let steep, covered, for 10 minutes, then strain. Add the extract to the bath water.

Temperature of bath water, 98.6°F (37°C); length of bath, ten minutes. Rest after bathing.

● **Spruce needle bath**

Pour 5 quarts (5 L) of water over 3.52 ounces (100 g) of fresh spruce needles, bring to a boil, let steep for ten minutes, then strain. Add the extract to the bath water.

Temperature of bath water, 98.6°F (37°C); length of bath, ten minutes. Rest after bathing.

● **Hayseed bath**

Pour 5 quarts (5 L) of water over 10.58 to 17.63 ounces (300–500 g) of hayseed, bring to a boil, let boil about 15 minutes, then strain. Add the extract to the bath water.

Temperature of bath water, 98.6°F (37°C); length of bath, 10 to 15 minutes. Rest after bathing.

● **Lemon balm bath**

Pour 5 quarts (5 L) of boiling water over 2.11 to 2.46 ounces (60–70 g) of lemon balm leaves, let steep about 20 minutes, then strain. Add the extract to the bath water.

Temperature of bath water, 95 to 100.4°F (35–38°C); length of bath, 10 to 15 minutes. Rest after bathing.

● **Thyme bath**

Pour 3 quarts (3 L) of water over 3.52 ounces (100 g) of thyme (aerial parts), bring to a boil, let steep, covered, about 20 minutes, then strain. Add the extract to the bath water.

Temperature of bath water, 95 to 100.4°F (35–38°C); length of bath, 10 to 15 minutes. Rest after bathing.

If it is too tedious to prepare your bath additive yourself, buy ready-made ones (pharmacy or health food store). It is important, however, to differentiate between purely cosmetic baths and medicinal baths; you need to make sure that the essential oils from the herbs are contained in sufficient quantities in the bath additive.

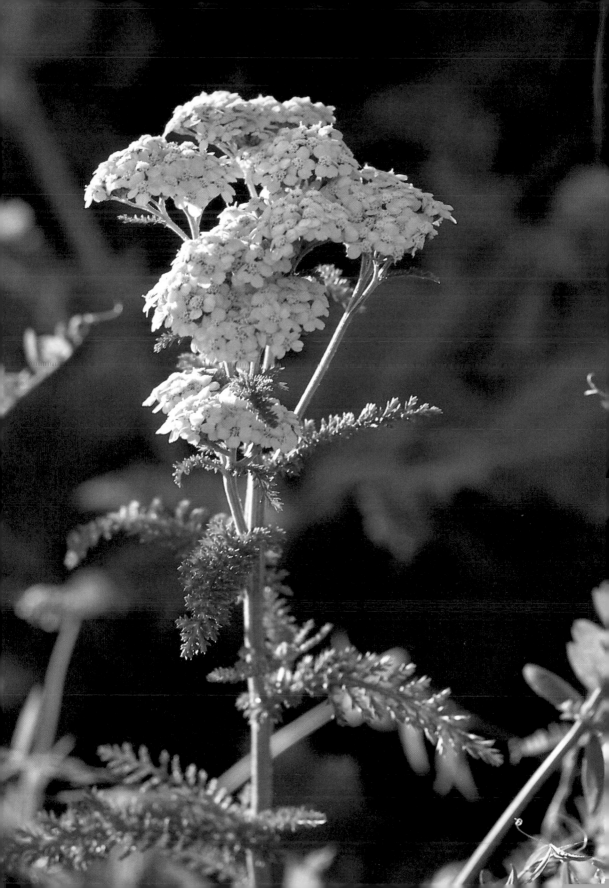

Bladder and Kidney Complaints

← *Yarrow*

Self-treatment—Only in Cooperation with Your Physician!

Only in a few cases can you treat bladder and kidney complaints yourself, because there is great danger that a layman will incorrectly diagnose the problem or overlook serious disorders. This means that working together with your physician is essential if you are suffering from bladder or kidney trouble! Be sure to observe the limits of self-treatment (see page 7), and these pointers in particular:

Please note
Go to the doctor immediately if the following symptoms appear:
● Cramplike pain in the kidney area or in the bladder region, accompanied by high fever.
● If you wake up in the mornings with swollen eyelids.
● If you experience extreme thirst and fatigue and your complexion becomes pallid.
● If your urine is cloudy, reddish, or red in color, or if urination is painful.

I strongly advise older men who are having trouble urinating—even though they may experience no pain—to see a physician. The probable cause is the prostate gland, which in most men undergoes benign enlargement (hyperplasia or BPH) as they age and obstructs the flow of urine (see page 122). Nevertheless, this has to be clarified by a physician, as malignant tumors of the prostate begin with the very same (initially painless) symptoms.

Medicinal Plants Support the Doctor's Therapy

Many physicians do not reject phytotherapy (treatment with medicinal herbs or with medications made from them) for bladder and kidney disorders. In the treatment of benign prostate trouble (see page 49), bed-wetting (see page 94), or an irritable bladder, medicinal plants are also indispensable aids.

From the great number of effective medicinal plants I have selected for you those that are reliable and are sometimes used by physicians.

Bladder Complaints

Acute Bladder Infection (Cystitis)

The factors that generally trigger an acute bladder infection are cold and dampness. Cold feet, wet bathing suits in summer that are not removed immediately after swimming, drafts, or sitting on cold ground for a prolonged time weaken the body's powers of resistance. As a result, the pathogens that have made their way into the bladder have an opportunity to become active.

For Prevention

● **Warm clothing**
Make sure you always wear warm clothing, keep your feet and hands warm, and—if possible—wear an undershirt at all times.

● **Progressively hot footbath**
If you ever have cold or, even worse, clammy feet, immediately take a progressively hot footbath with a horsetail or hayseed (see page 39) additive. If you have a "weak" bladder; that is, if you suffer frequently from nonspecific acute bladder infections, take special note of these pointers.

● **Horsetail bath**
According to the recommendations of home remedies, all young girls and women who have a "weak bladder" should take a horsetail bath twice a week, in the form of a sitz bath or, preferably, a full bath (see page 14). This strengthens the weak bladder and prevents disease.

● **Hygienic measures**
Girls and women in particular frequently suffer from nonspecific acute bladder infections. In over 50 percent of the cases the pathogens are intestinal bacteria that "migrate" via the urethra. Because the urethra is much shorter in women than in men, women are at far greater risk. They can, however, prevent bladder infection through hygienic measures, by making it a habit after a bowel movement to direct the toilet paper toward the buttocks and away from the vagina.

● **Improved emptying of the bladder**
In men, cystitis also can be caused by failure to empty the bladder completely, due to pathological changes in the prostate. Some urine remains in the bladder after voiding, and this residue frequently becomes a breeding ground for bacteria.

To increase urination, two medicinal plants have proved valuable: stinging nettle and dandelion. They strengthen the muscle tone of the bladder, thus reducing the amount of residual urine. After a course of treatment (three to six weeks) with the following tea blend, voiding will return to normal again. The improvement generally is long-lived.

Tea Blend	oz. (g)
Stinging nettle leaves	.88 (25)
Stinging nettle roots	.88 (25)
Dandelion roots (with	
aerial parts)	.88 (25)

Preparation: Pour 8 ounces (1/4 L) of cold water over 2 heaping teaspoonfuls of this mixture, slowly bring to a boil, let steep for three to five minutes, then strain.
Application: Drink three to five cups per day.

Burning During Urination

An acute bladder infection usually begins suddenly with intense pain during urination and a constant urge to urinate, accompanied by a burning sensation, especially at the conclusion of micturition (urination). Fever usually is not present.

Please note
Go to the doctor immediately if you have fever.

● **Bearberry leaf tea**

A tea made from bearberry leaves usually brings swift relief. When preparing it, keep the following in mind: Bearberry leaves are quite high in tannin, which places a strain on the stomach and may trigger unpleasant side effects such as nausea and vomiting. For this reason, the cold method of preparation has to be used; in this way, only a fraction of the tannins, but almost all the active substances, are extracted.

Tea blends that contain bearberry leaves, however, need not be prepared by the cold method.

Preparation: Pour 8 ounces (1/4 L) of room-temperature water over 2 heaping teaspoonfuls of bearberry leaves, let steep, stirring frequently, for five to six hours, then warm to drinking temperature.

Application: Drink three to five cups of tea daily.

Bearberry tea, however, is effective only if the urine has an alkaline reaction; only then will the arbutene split off disinfectant hydroquinone. This can be accomplished by adding to every cup of tea one large pinch of bicarbonate of soda, or over the long run, by eating a predominantly vegetable diet.

● **Tea blend**

In treating cystitis, a blend of the following ingredients has also proved useful, instead of bearberry leaf tea:

Bearberry leaves	1.05 (30)
Chamomile flowers	.70 (20)
Orthosiphon leaves	.35 (10)
Herniary, aerial parts	.35 (10)

Preparation, see page 14.

Application: Drink five cups of tea per day, adding one large pinch of bicarbonate of soda to each.

Please note

Go to the doctor if the problems continue for more than two or three days! In this case, the doctor will have to employ stronger remedies.

Follow-up Treatment for Cystitis

Once you have gotten over the acute phase, follow-up treatment of cystitis is recommended. Drink plenty of tea (1 to 2 quarts [1–2 L] daily!) to flush the bacteria completely out of the bladder. The tea should have a diuretic (promoting and increasing urine flow) effect, which is undesirable in the acute stage.

● **Tea blends**

Several tea blends, all with similar effects but different tastes, are available for this purpose. Try them and see which blend tastes best.

Tea Blend 1

Dandelion roots (with leaves)	.70 (20)
Field horsetail, aerial parts	.35 (10)
Rose hips (with seeds)	.35 (10)
Peppermint leaves	.35 (10)

Tea Blend 2

Birch leaves	.70 (20)
Orthosiphon leaves	.70 (20)
Fennel seeds/crushed)	.35 (10)
Chamomile flowers	.35 (10)
Licorice root	.35 (10)

Tea Blend 3

Goldenrod, aerial parts	.70 (20)
Bean hulls (without seeds)	.35 (10)
Stinging nettle leaves	.35 (10)
Peppermint leaves	.35 (10)
Elderberry flowers	.35 (10)

Preparation: Pour 1 quart (1 L) of boiling water over 3 tablespoonfuls of the blend in question, let steep, covered, for five minutes, then strain.

Application: Several times between meals drink a cup of tea, at least 1 quart (1 L) during the course of the day. Sweetening with honey is beneficial (diabetics should not sweeten).

Chronic Bladder Infection

Quadriplegics often suffer from chronic bladder infection or recurring cystitis.

● **Tea blend**
Here you can use a tea blend containing equal parts of the following:

Chamomile flowers
Bearberry leaves
Herniary, aerial part

Preparation, see page 14.
Application: Drink three to five cups of tea per day.

Bladder and Kidney Stones, Gravel

Urinary calculus is one of the most common diseases. Although it is not a "new" disease (we have reason to believe that it is as old as mankind), this malady has increased markedly in recent years. We attribute this alarmingly large increase to changes in life-style. We eat more protein in the form of meat, we get less exercise, and we are gaining weight.

Urinary calculus (a comprehensive term for uroliths, or stones, in the kidney, ureter, or bladder, whatever their composition) is produced whenever salts crystallize out of the urine and mass together to form solid structures (concretions). Only a tiny percentage of urinary calculus causes problems. Many stones remain lying in the kidney unbeknownst to the person affected; smaller stones are passed without causing pain. Only when a larger stone is washed into the ureter and gets stuck there does colic pain result. The ureter tries to "pass" the stone, which, depending on the size of the urolith, causes such excruciating pain that the doctor has to inject powerful painkillers. This pain usually originates in the kidney area and radiates into the abdominal area, even into the thighs. The sufferers writhe in agony; they often feel queasy and are troubled by severe nausea.

Please note
Painful though kidney and bladder colics may be, they are not fatal. In any event, however, you should see a doctor immediately after an attack of kidney or bladder colic! The urine voided during or after the colic needs to be collected—first, to check whether the stone has been expelled, second, to have the discharged stone examined to determine its composition.

Uroliths differ in terms of their components. They consist of uric acid, cystine, oxalate, phosphate, or calcium. Frequently they are mixtures of all these ingredients. Their structure tells the doctor whether there is any chance of dissolving the stones.

Help from Medicinal Plants

If the stone has been discharged, calm descends once more. If it has become stuck in the ureter, it has to be removed, so that the flow of urine can proceed unimpeded. Over two-thirds of all uroliths are discharged on their own, with the aid of some additional measures. Teas made from medicinal plants are extremely helpful.

First, however, it is important to deal with colics in their initial stage and to alleviate the pain already present, so that the doctor does not need to inject strong painkillers.

Relief of Pain Caused by Colic

● **Chamomile tea**

If used promptly, hot chamomile tea (*Preparation*, see page 14), through its spasmolytic (antispasmodic) effect, can make it easier for the stone to move in the ureter and thus to be expelled.

● **Tea blends**

There are, however, other herbal spasmolytics, such as peppermint leaves, fennel seeds, the aerial parts of herniary, lemon balm leaves, the aerial parts of yarrow, or coriander seeds, that are helpful when a colic begins.

Tea Blend 1

Chamomile flowers	.35 (10)
Peppermint leaves	.35 (10)
Lemon balm leaves	.35 (10)
Herniary, aerial parts	.35 (10)
Coriander seeds	.17 (5)
Yarrow, aerial parts	.17 (5)

Preparation, see page 14.
Application: With colics, drink one or two cups of tea, as hot as possible.

Tea Blend 2

Also helpful is a tea blend containing European centaury (aerial parts), peppermint leaves, chamomile flowers, and lemon balm leaves in equal parts.

Preparation, see page 14.
Application: With colics, drink one cup of tea, as hot as possible.

The tonic (strengthening) effect of the bitter constituent present in European centaury speaks for the use of this herb. That effect makes it easier for the ureter to get rid of the stone.

● **Hayseed poultice and bath**

Hot baths and hot poultices can also ease the pain of colics.

Hayseed (see page 174) has the most powerful effect. A hayseed bath (see pages 25 and 39) in 100.4°F (38°C) water can bring marked relief; the hayseed poultice, or hayseed bag, is reputedly even more effective. (Flaxseed poultices are also very helpful.)

Preparation and application of a hayseed poultice: You need a coarse linen bag the size of the area to be treated. Fill this bag about 2 to 3 inches (5–8 cm) deep with hayseed, put it in a pot, pour boiling water over it, and let it steep for 15 minutes. Then squeeze the water out of the bag, ideally by pressing it between two boards. Change the position of the bag and repeat the procedure to force out as much liquid as possible. Wrap the hayseed poultice thus prepared in a cloth and lay it on the painful body area that needs treatment. The poultice should lie flat, without wrinkles. Hold it in place with another cloth or an elastic bandage. The temperature of the poultice should be about 107.6°F (42°C), and the treatment should last about 30 minutes.

A second method of preparing the hayseed poultice is steaming it. For this you need a pot with a rack that fits inside (a large kettle used for canning, for example). Put some water in the pot and place the poultice on the rack. The water should not be deep enough to touch the poultice. Now heat the water to the boiling point. The rising steam will penetrate the hayseed and heat and moisten it sufficiently. This will take about 10 minutes. Then the hayseed poultice will be ready to use, and there will be no need to squeeze it out.

Expelling Kidney Stones

● Massive dose of water

Once things have calmed down after the colic, a massive dose of water may succeed in dislodging a stone that has not been discharged.

> **Please note**
> An application of this kind, of course, first has to be coordinated with your doctor. Doctors who are partial to naturopathy welcome such measures and recommend them to their patients.

For the massive dose of water, drink a large amount of tea made from diuretic herbs. This will produce a mighty flood of urine, which will loosen the stones and carry them out of the body.

Suitable for use as diuretic tea herbs are, above all, dandelion (roots plus aerial parts), goldenrod (aerial parts), field horsetail (aerial parts), and birch leaves. My preference is dandelion tea.

Preparation and application: Pour 1 quart (1 L) of boiling water over 3 tablespoonfuls of dandelion roots and aerial parts, let steep for ten minutes, then strain. Next, dilute this tea with 8 ounces (1/4 L) of lukewarm water. Drink the entire amount—some 1-1/4 quarts (1-1/4 L) as quickly as possible. After a few minutes a flood of urine will begin, which will allow the stones still present to "pass" (to check this, collect and strain the urine).

Preventing the Formation of Stones

Anyone who has been through a severe stone colic will be bent on ensuring that it does not happen again. Basically, however, it makes sense for everyone, through preventive behavior, to forestall the formation of stones.

● Drink plenty of liquids

The first commandment is: Drink plenty of liquids! Salts can crystallize only from concentrated urine. Drink at least 2 quarts (2 L) of fluids per day. Actually these can be any fluids, apart from alcoholic beverages and sugary soft drinks. Milk, however, is also not recommended in such quantities.

If you ensure a "lively" flow of urine, you also will irrigate the kidneys thoroughly and at the same time prevent other diseases (infections).

● Tea blends

All medicinal herbs classified as diuretics are suitable for this purpose. They increase urine production. Among many possibilities, I have chosen those medicinal plants that have proved reliable in practice.

I can recommend dandelion roots along with the aerial parts, birch leaves, orthosiphon leaves (Indian bladder and kidney tea), the aerial parts of goldenrod, stinging nettle leaves, the aerial parts of field horsetail, and bean hulls without seeds.

I cannot recommend juniper berries, a favorite in folk medicine, and parsley root, as both irritate kidney tissue if used for a prolonged period.

Because such teas need to be used over a long period to have a prophylactic (preventive) effect, the single teas should be drunk in rotation. Mixing the medicinal herbs together is even better, so that the assortment of teas available will have as much variety as possible. In contrast to medicinal teas intended for short-term use, these irrigating teas may by all means be combined with other herbs that may not be particularly diuretic but do taste good.

Here, some suggestions for you to try:

Tea Blend 1

Dandelion roots (with aerial parts)	.70 (20)
Birch leaves	.70 (20)
Stinging nettle leaves	.70 (20)
Rose hips (with seeds)	.70 (20)
Chamomile flowers	.70 (20)

Tea Blend 2

Orthosiphon leaves	.70 (20)
Goldenrod, aerial parts	.70 (20)
Field horsetail, aerial parts	.70 (20)
Peppermint leaves	.35 (10)
Bean hulls (without seeds)	.35 (10)

Tea Blend 3

Field horsetail, aerial parts	.70 (20)
Goldenrod, aerial parts	.70 (20)
Dandelion roots (with aerial parts)	.70 (20)
Lemon balm leaves	.35 (10)
Peppermint leaves	.35 (10)
Hibiscus flowers	.35 (10)

Tea Blend 4

Stinging nettle leaves	.70 (20)
Goldenrod, aerial parts	.70 (20)
Chamomile flowers	.70 (20)
Raspberry leaves	.70 (20)
Strawberry leaves	.70 (20)

Tea Blend 5

Dandelion roots (with aerial parts)	.70 (20)
Orthosiphon leaves	.70 (20)
Birch leaves	.70 (20)
Stinging nettle leaves	.70 (20)
Peppermint leaves	.35 (10)
Bitter-orange peel	.35 (10)

Preparation of these tea blends: Pour 1 quart (1 L) of boiling water over 3 tablespoonfuls of the blend selected, let steep for five to ten minutes, then strain.

Application: Several times a day between meals, drink one cup of tea (2 quarts [2 L] per day).

● **Madder root**

In our great-great-grandmothers' day, madder root (the root of dyer's madder) played quite a role as a remedy for kidney and bladder stones, but thereafter little more was heard about it. Just as madder dye, once used to impart color to fabrics (French soldiers' red trousers, for example), was replaced by aniline dyes, modern chemical agents supplanted madder root as a medicine—until people came back to it again because little

progress had been made in the treatment and prevention of urinary calculi.

The substances contained in madder root, especially ruberythrine acid, reduce the calcium and magnesium ions present in slightly acid urine and thus interfere with the formation of stones. Because urinary stones are not exclusively calcium stones, however, madder root is not effective in countering all stone formation. There is reason to suspect, though, that even hybrid stones can be "split up."

Tea made from madder root has quite an unpleasant taste, and it would be pointless to offer a recipe here. The powdered root, however, can be taken in wafer form, and it is worth recommending.

Please note
Madder root is difficult to obtain. Further, a course of treatment with powdered madder root may be carried out only under medical supervision!

Organic Bladder Disorders

Irritable Bladder

Middle-aged women—to a markedly lesser extent once they pass the age of sixty—frequently suffer from problems that closely resemble an acute bladder infection, but without any pathological findings upon medical examination. The women affected are greatly bothered by an intense, frequent need to urinate. If they go to the toilet, they are able to void only a small amount of urine. These problems are functional bladder disorders, such as poor tone in the bladder muscles.

An irritable bladder is difficult to treat with medications. As a result, increased attention is now being paid to tea therapy.

Strengthening the Nervous System

What is called for here is not the healing plants used for bladder and kidney complaints, but others that can stabilize the autonomic nervous system and that have tonic (strengthening) properties. European centaury, St. John's wort, hop cones, lemon balm, valerian, and chamomile can be helpful here.

● **Tea blends**
The following tea blends deserve at least a try:

Tea Blend 1

St. John's wort, aerial parts	.70 (20)
Lemon balm leaves	.70 (20)
Chamomile flowers	.70 (20)
European centaury, aerial parts	.35 (10)
Rose hips (with seeds)	.35 (10)
Hop cones	.17 (5)

Tea Blend 2

Lemon balm leaves	.70 (20)
Chamomile flowers	.70 (20)
Valerian roots	.70 (20)

Tea Blend 3

Lemon balm leaves	.35 (10)
Peppermint leaves	.35 (10)
Lavender flowers	.35 (10)
Orange flowers	.35 (10)
Bitter-orange peel	.35 (10)
Valerian roots	.35 (10)

Preparation of these tea blends: Pour 8 ounces (1/4 L) of boiling water over 2 to 3 heaping tablespoonfuls of the tea in question, let steep for about ten minutes, then strain.

Application: Drink two to three cups of tea daily. Sweetening with honey is advisable (diabetics do not sweeten).

● **Herbal baths**
Medicinal herbal baths support the treatment. Appropriate here are lemon balm baths, yarrow baths, and lavender flower baths (see page 25), in the form of either full or partial baths. Highly recommended as well are hayseed baths (see page 25) and hayseed poultices (see page 46).

● **Homeopathic remedies**
A recommended remedy is *Sabal Serrulata* (derived from the saw palm, or dwarf palm, native to the southern part of North America) in the second (2x), fourth (4x), or sixth (6x) decimal potency. Take 5 drops two to three times daily.

● **General rules of behavior**
In conclusion, a word about general rules of behavior. If you have an irritable bladder, dress warmly, though not too warmly, keep your feet dry and warm, avoid stimulants (coffee, cigarettes, alcohol) or use them sparingly, and try to get enough sleep and to plan a daily routine devoid of hustle and bustle.

Prostate Neurosis

Prostate neurosis has about the same effect as an irritable bladder in women: an unnatural need to urinate, although the bladder is not full. As medical examination reveals, it is not a question of an inflamed prostate (see also page 121), but of a functional disorder, an imbalance between the reaction of the sphincter and the muscle that brings about the voiding of urine. If the bladder muscles in general are also weakened, the complaints described above can result.

The medicinal plants required for therapy are those that stabilize the autonomic nervous system and those with tonic properties. They are the same plants used to treat irritable bladder in women: European centaury, St. John's wort, hop cones, lemon balm, valerian, and chamomile. For this reason, I suggest that you try the tea blends recommended on page 49.

Preparation and application are the same. The homeopathic remedy presented there, *Sabal Serrulata*, is also helpful, as is a plain, hot water sitz bath. In conclusion, let me refer you again to the general rules of behavior at the end of the previous section (see page 49), which also apply in cases of prostate neurosis.

Additional Remedies for Bladder and Kidney Complaints

Herbal Baths to Calm and Relax

Several herbal baths, some of which I have recommended in the applications contained in this chapter, will help ease your pain—try them and see which works best for you.

The quantities given are sufficient for one full bath.

How to prepare the herbal baths:

● **Oat straw bath**
(calms)
Pour 3 to 5 quarts (3–5 L) of water over 3.52 to 5.29 ounces (100–150 g) of cut-up (chopped) oat straw (for partial baths, 1.76 ounces [50 g] will suffice), bring to a boil, let boil for about 20 minutes, then strain. Add the extract to the bath water.

Temperature of bath water, 95 to 100.4°F (35–38°C), length of bath, 10 to 15 minutes. Rest after bathing.

● **Hayseed bath**
(relaxes, relieves pain, calms)
Pour 5 quarts (5 L) of water over 10.58 to 17.63 ounces (300–500 g) of hayseed (for partial baths, 5.29 ounces [150 g] will suffice), bring to a boil, let boil for about 15 minutes, then strain. Add the extract to the bath water.

Temperature of bath water, 95 to 100.4°F (35–38°C), length of bath, 10 to 15 minutes. Rest after bathing.

● **Chamomile bath**
(relaxes, relieves pain, calms, disinfects)
One tablespoonful of chamomile flowers per quart (1 L) of water is required. Pour 2 to 5 quarts (2–5 L) of boiling water over the chamomile flowers, let steep for 15 minutes, then strain. Add the extract to the bath water.

Temperature of bath water, 95 to 100.4°F (35–38°C), length of bath, 10 to 15 minutes. Rest after bathing.

● **Lavender flower bath**
(calms)
Pour 5 quarts (5 L) of boiling water over 2.11 to 2.46 ounces (60–70 g) of lavender flowers, let steep about 20 minutes, then strain. Add the extract to the bath water.
Temperature of bath water, 95 to 100.4°F (35–38°C), length of bath, 10 to 15 minutes. Rest after bathing.

● **Lemon balm bath**
(calms, soothes)
Pour 5 quarts (5 L) of boiling water over 2.11 to 2.46 ounces (60–70 g) of lemon balm leaves, let steep for about 20 minutes, then strain. Add the extract to the bath water.
Temperature of bath water, 95 to 100.4°F (35–38°C), length of bath, 10 to 15 minutes. Rest after bathing.

● **Yarrow bath**
(calms, relaxes, disinfects)
Pour 5 quarts (5 L) of boiling water over 2.11 to 2.46 ounces (60–70 g) of yarrow (aerial parts), let steep for about 20 minutes, then strain. Add the extract to the bath water.
Temperature of bath water, 95 to 100.4°F (35–38°C), length of bath, 10 to 15 minutes. Rest after bathing.

● **Field horsetail bath**
(especially recommended for bladder and kidneys)
Soak 3.52 to 5.29 ounces (100–150 g) of the aerial parts of field horsetail (for partial baths, 1.76 ounces [50 g] will suffice) in 2 to 3 quarts (2–3 L) of hot water for about one hour, then bring briefly to a boil and strain. Add the extract to the bath water.
Temperature of bath water, 95 to 100.4°F (35–38°C), length of bath, 10 to 15 minutes. Rest after bathing.

If it is too troublesome to prepare your own bath additive, it is sometimes possible to buy ready-made ones (in pharmacies). It is important, however, to distinguish between purely cosmetic baths and medicinal baths; you need to make sure that the essential oils or the other active substances are present in sufficient quantities in the bath additives.

Blood-cleansing Treatments for Purification

Here we refer to the courses of treatment undertaken in fall and spring, generally known and loved by the name of "blood-purifying cures." Their purpose is to "toughen" from the inside, to activate body metabolism, to achieve an alterative effect, and to purify. People use them also to increase their level of vitality and to feel fresher and healthier.

Perhaps you are wondering what treatments of this kind have to do with the topic of bladder and kidney complaints. The most important plants used in treating these complaints also form the basis of the blood-purifying teas. Without birch leaves, dandelion roots, the aerial parts of goldenrod and field horsetail, stinging nettle leaves, or chamomile flowers, the traditional blood-cleansing teas are scarcely conceivable.

Further, these teas contain medicinal plants with tonic (strengthening) bitter constituents or aromatic substances, such as the aerial parts of European centaury, mugwort, or wormwood, bitter-orange peel, and peppermint or lemon balm leaves, as well as other medicinal plants that are considered to be metabolic remedies, such as elderberry flowers, eyebright (aerial parts), couch grass roots, or wild pansies (aerial parts), to name only a few. Lavender flowers, rose hips with seeds, hibiscus flowers, and orange flowers are used to improve the taste. A spot of color is provided by red sandalwood, yellow pussy-toes or yellow pot marigold petals, and blue cornflowers.

In this list you may notice the absence of purgative medicinal herbs like senna seedpods, senna leaves, European alder-buckthorn bark, or

51

rhubarb roots. However: A blood-purifying tea is not a laxative tea! In earlier times the negative effect of these medicinal plants was not known, and it was believed that drastic "scouring" (purging) was good and useful. Today, however, we reserve the laxative drugs listed above for short-term treatment of acute constipation, or we resort to their use only when a physician has specified soft bowel movements. If the drugs are used for long periods, the body loses important minerals or is made ill by continued irritation of the large intestine.

The once so popular juniper berries, which at one time were a component of every depurative tea, also have been excluded here, because they irritate the kidneys, at least with sustained use. In addition, they are not good for pregnant women and nursing mothers, and they easily can be replaced with other diuretic medicinal plants.

● **Tea blends**

If properly constituted, blood-purifying teas are healthful house teas. Used in a course of treatment, they strengthen the body's ability to heal itself. In addition, they activate all its metabolic processes.

Below are several well-tested recipes for spring and fall "cures":

Tea Blend 1

Birch leaves	.35 (10)
Stinging nettle leaves	.35 (10)
Rose hips (with seeds)	.35 (10)
Goldenrod, aerial parts	.35 (10)
Dandelion roots (with aerial parts)	.35 (10)
Pot marigold flowers	.17 (5)
Red sandalwood	.17 (5)
Pussy-toes	.17 (5)
Peppermint leaves	.17 (5)

Tea Blend 2

Elderberry leaves	.35 (10)
Field horsetail, aerial parts	.35 (10)
Bean hulls	35 (10)
Stinging nettle leaves	.35 (10)
Bitter-orange peel	.17 (5)
European centaury, aerial parts	.17 (5)

Tea Blend 3

Mugwort, aerial parts	.35 (10)
Raspberry leaves	.35 (10)
Chamomile flowers	.35 (10)
Birch leaves	.35 (10)
Goldenrod, aerial parts	.35 (10)
Hibiscus flowers	.35 (10)
Elderberry flowers	.35 (10)
Linden flowers	.35 (10)

Tea Blend 4

Pansies, aerial parts	.35 (10)
Eyebright, aerial parts	.35 (10)
Elderberry flower	.35 (10)
Dandelion roots (with aerial parts)	.35 (10)
Lavender flowers	.17 (5)
Lemon balm leaves	.17 (5)
Peppermint leaves	.17 (5)
Birch leaves	.17 (5)
Rose hips (without seeds)	.17 (5)

Tea Blend 5

(slightly laxative in effect; for this reason, do not use longer than two to three weeks!)

Fennel seeds (crushed)	.35 (10)
European alder-buckthorn bark	.35 (10)
Senna seedpods (fruits)	.35 (10)
Rose hips (with seeds)	.17 (5)
Hibiscus flowers	.17 (5)
Orange flowers	.17 (5)
Birch leaves	.17 (5)
Goldenrod, aerial parts	.17 (5)
European centaury, aerial parts	.17 (5)
Strawberry leaves	.52 (15)
Raspberry leaves	.52 (15)
Blackberry leaves	.52 (15)

Preparation of these tea blends: Pour 8 ounces (1/4 L) of boiling water over 2 heaping teaspoonfuls of the blend in question, let steep, covered, for 10 minutes, then strain.

Application: Drink one cup of tea two to five times daily. With the exception of Blend 5, all the teas recommended can be used in a course of treatment lasting four to six weeks.

Blend 5, owing to its mildly laxative effect, may be drunk for only two to three weeks!

Bladder and Kidney Teas

Bladder diseases and, above all, kidney diseases are a serious matter and can be treated only by a physician. Naturally we have to wonder about the value of the many bladder and kidney teas available commercially.

If you look at the ingredients of the bladder and kidney teas on the market, you will see that they are mixtures of medicinal herbs that have a disinfectant effect (bearberry leaves, orthosiphon leaves), antispasmodic properties (for example, chamomile flowers, the aerial parts of herniary, peppermint leaves), and, above all, a diuretic effect (the aerial parts of goldenrod, birch leaves, dandelion roots with the aerial parts, the aerial parts of field horsetail). They are used as accompanying therapy for medical treatment of bladder and kidney complaints; they disinfect and irrigate the urinary passages; and they can be enlisted for long-term treatment of chronic bladder and kidney problems. They also help keep the bladder and kidneys healthy.

A tea blend containing birch leaves, bearberry leaves, dandelion roots, rose hips, the aerial parts of goldenrod, and hibiscus flowers is available in health food stores. It is particularly recommended if your doctor suggests irrigation therapy to treat existing bacteriuria (bacteria in the urine).

There are also instant teas available for people who are always in a hurry.

Please note
Go to your doctor immediately if you have bladder or kidney problems. Discuss with him or her which medicinal plant applications are advisable as an adjunct to the medical therapy.

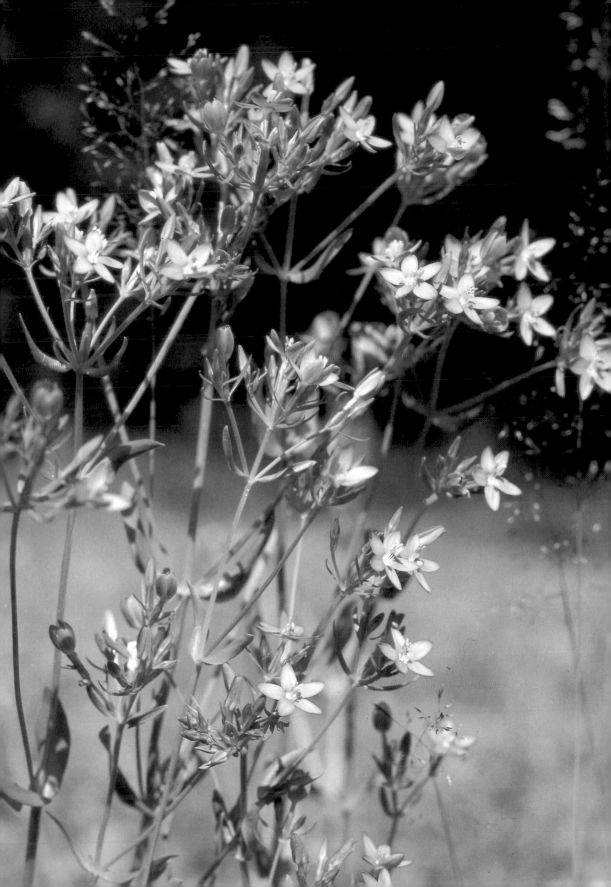

Stomach and Intestinal Complaints

← *European centaury*

Medicinal Plants That Act on the Stomach

If you ever have occasion to look at old and more recent books of folk medicine dealing with medicinal herbs or to leaf through old volumes of household remedies, you will notice that the number of plants used for stomach and intestinal complaints is almost indeterminable. The range extends from anise to zubrovka, from native to European, African, or East Asian medicinal plants. These healing plants either taste bitter, acrid, or aromatic or have a high mucilage content.

In all, far more than 100 different medicinal plants are used in treating gastrointestinal conditions. For this reason you will be surprised and amazed that I am recommending only a few of them for your use in the treatment of such complaints. These few, however, are the ones with which I have had outstanding success over decades of experience and whose effect has been validated by scientific research; in other words, medicinal plants on which you can rely.

First on my list are the medicinal plants that taste bitter and aromatic, the *Amara* (for example, gentian roots and the aerial parts of European centaury) and the *Amara aromatica* (for example, bitter-orange peel, wormwood, and mugwort). Then come the medicinal plants that taste acrid or acrid and aromatic, the *Acria* (for example, paprika) or *Acria aromatica* (for example, ginger). Bitter and acrid substances step up the activity of the digestive juices, thus stimulating the appetite and making "heavy" foods easier to digest.

Many medicinal plants that act on the stomach also contain essential oils (the odoriferous substances of the plants); they support the effect of the bitter and acrid substances. Moreover, essential oils are antispasmodic or calming and anti-inflammatory (for example, the essential oils found in lemon balm and chamomile).

Caraway, coriander, and fennel, through their essential oils, have a special effect—they help relieve cramps and gas pains (that is, they are spasmolytic and carminative).

Medicinal plants that contain tannins—erect cinquefoil, for example—are useful to combat diarrhea. Plants such as senna and European alder-buckthorn, which contain laxative anthraquinones, are good remedies for constipation.

Mucilage-containing plants, such as flax, protect the irritated gastrointestinal mucous membranes and are slightly laxative, because the mucins swell in the intestinal tract and also act as lubricants. In the case of flax, this effect is due to the fat content.

Season with Medicinal Plants—Ease Discomfort

We generally use herbs and spices to improve the smell and taste of our food, yet—if properly employed—they can accomplish far more. For example, use of hearty seasonings is often sufficient to prevent indispositions in the gastrointestinal area. In particular, older people with chronic digestive problems are helped by proper seasoning of their foods to enjoy improved digestion. Long ago it was scientifically proved that herbs and spices can stimulate the appetite or make the digestion of food easier, because they activate the glands that produce gastric juice. In addition, they can lessen the strain on the heart and circulatory system.

Spicy seasonings in particular intensify the progress of almost all vital processes, which results in increased vitality. If you want an all-around feeling of well-being, frequently add spicy seasonings like paprika, cayenne pepper, ginger, mustard, or turmeric to your foods. Through proper seasoning you can substantially improve your general health. For this purpose, the amount of seasoning that suits your taste is usually sufficient.

In Mexico, where people enjoy eating fiery chili peppers, and in the Balkans, where hot paprika is popular, fewer people suffer heart attacks than in this country. As research over time has revealed, the spices used are partially responsible for this.

We also know that seasonings have specific effects: Cloves, for example, known in the kitchen only as an aromatic spice, aid in the healing of stomach ulcers.

Before the positive effect of seasonings on our health could be proved, it was considered nutritionally incorrect for older people or people with gastrointestinal problems to season their foods heartily—a bland diet was recommended. The opposite is true, however: Spicy and bitter seasonings stimulate the "animal spirits."

Following is a list of reliable seasonings and culinary herbs to which you should give preference in treating certain gastrointestinal disturbances. Some of them you can easily raise yourself in a garden or in balcony boxes (see page 138).

Weak Stomach

Do you have the unpleasant feeling that your stomach is not emptying properly, because food "lies like a rock" in your stomach? Do you have a sensation of pressure after meals? Use these herbs as seasonings frequently: mugwort, wormwood, basil, summer savory, marjoram, and thyme.

These seasonings also have proved suitable: mustard, paprika, nutmeg, ginger, and hot curry.

Please note the following rule: The fattier the foods, the more heartily you should season them.

Lack of Appetite

Do you pick at your food reluctantly or sit at the table with no desire to eat and no enjoyment? You can stimulate your appetite again with the following herbs and spices: cayenne pepper, hot mustard (moderately hot to hot prepared mustard), ginger, and thyme.

Feeling of Fullness and Flatulence

Do you regularly suffer from a sensation of fullness and gas pains after eating? Above all, when you have eaten fresh bread, legumes, vegetable soup, vegetable stew, or cabbage? I recommend that you try caraway and coriander, because these seasonings will mitigate or even prevent both abdominal fullness and flatulence.

If your problems are mild in nature, you may even get relief from milder seasonings like anise and fennel.

Flatulence Accompanied by Diarrhea

Do you suffer from flatulence in combination with foamy, foul-smelling diarrhea? These problems appear when food begins to ferment in the stomach. A great number of herbs and spices can be helpful here:

Especially efficacious are garlic and radish. Summer savory, marjoram, lemon balm, pepper mint, and thyme, also have proved effective.

For a Nervous Stomach

Do you have the feeling that your stomach hasn't "processed" the food properly, because your nervous tension has "upset your stomach?" Then you should begin every meal with a fragrant soup, for example, bouillon or vegetable soup. Use fresh herbs to season the soup just before serving: dill weed, lemon balm leaves, and basil.

For your main meal, the appropriate herbs and spices are basil, lemon balm, mugwort, and mustard (prepared mustard)

Please be courageous— experiment with herbs and spices in your kitchen. Perhaps proper seasoning alone will be enough to get rid of your gastrointestinal discomfort. In any event, support your other efforts to improve your health with generous use of the right herbs and spices.

Seasoning properly also means leading a healthier life.

Symptoms and Their Treatment

The Overloaded Stomach

An overloaded stomach is no rarity, because when food tastes good, we often don't know when we have eaten enough.

Adults overload their stomachs frequently—when they eat overly heavy (fatty) foods, drink alcoholic beverages, or smoke. The consequence is an acute irritation of the gastric mucous membranes. Nausea and vomiting, a feeling of pressure, or heartburn usually ensue.

Feeling of Pressure, Heartburn, Nausea

● **Tea blend**
A tea in which various medicinal herbs are blended is a time-tested remedy for these complaints:

	oz. (g)
Chamomile flowers	1.05 (30)
Lemon balm leaves	.35 (10)
Peppermint leaves	.35 (10)

Preparation, see page 14.

Application: Drink a total of three cups of tea, as warm as possible, at two-hour intervals. The acute problems should have vanished by then. What occasionally lingers is heartburn. If it still is bothering you the next day, chamomile tea will help (Preparation, see page 13). Sip one cup of it, as warm as possible, every two hours until the heartburn is gone.

● **Rolling After Drinking Chamomile Tea**
If your stomach upset is severe, try rolling, a method of treatment in which the patient drinks a liquid medication, then rotates his or her prone position every few minutes.

Preparation: The previous evening, prepare 8 ounces (1/4 L) of chamomile tea (*Preparation*, see page 14), pour it into a thermos bottle, and place it on your bedside table.

Implementation: The next morning, drink the tea as soon as you wake up. Then lie on your back, relaxed, for five minutes, followed by five minutes on your left side, then five minutes on your stomach, and finally five minutes on your right side. The rolling treatment is an effective remedy for acute stomach upsets. Don't worry that you will have to repeat the treatment over a prolonged period; one application provides all the help you need. This method, however, is frequently used in conservative treatment of stomach ulcers, in which case it is repeated over a period of four to six weeks.

Please note
If your physician has diagnosed a stomach ulcer, do not attempt self-treatment without consulting the doctor first! Medicinal plants with a high content of bitters are contra-indicated in this case.

The Irritable Stomach

What is meant by an irritable stomach, also known as a nervous stomach? It is not easy to describe. The complaints are diverse; they range from nervous agitation that also affects the gastrointestinal region through nausea to diarrhea and vomiting. Those afflicted suffer from a feeling of pressure in their abdomen and usually also from lack of appetite and a feeling of fullness after meals. In extreme cases the nervous stomach even causes cramplike pain.

Please note
These problems also can be symptoms of a serious illness. Be sure to respect the limits of self-treatment (see page 7).

It is usually people who are "overstressed" who suffer from a nervous stomach. Their daily life is hectic; they are no longer able to turn off their thoughts; they are afraid of failing in their career, of not getting their work done, or even of losing their job. Women whose triple load of running a household, raising children, and holding down a job "upsets their stomach" often suffer from these disorders. They have almost no free time, because they have to use the weekends to catch up on what didn't get done during the week. On vacation, then, many families long to "experience something special" at last and fly off on an adventure vacation or take an exhausting tour of other climate zones—which entails not relaxation, but increased stress.

For Prevention

The best way of preventing nervous indigestion is to regulate your daily routine so as to preclude any possibility of getting into a hectic state. This probably will not succeed right off the bat, but there are some effective methods that can help you find inner peace and tranquility (see Books for Further Reading, page 224).

It would be presumptuous to claim that medicinal herbal teas alone can bring quick relief to someone with a nervous stomach. Healing is possible only if you are prepared to make a change in your style of life, and this demands both patience and perseverance.

● **Organizing your life**
The first step required is to introduce order into your life. These suggestions may help you to do so:

Carefully separate your career from your private life. Work that you didn't finish at the office should not be brought home to do in your free time. Often, inefficient organization of time is responsible for not getting the job completed on office time—could this be your problem? Organize your work so that you can complete one task after another. If you start several tasks simultaneously, you can't finish any one of them properly—you will get into a frantic state, to which your stomach will react "irritably."

If ill feelings arise in dealing with coworkers, talk the situation out immediately and clear the air. This is just as important as any treatment with tea.

Don't start your evening in front of the television set; try to relax with a chat or a short walk—even if you get out just one stop earlier on your trip home and walk the last stretch of the way.

Before the evening meal, sip one cup of warm lemon balm tea (*Preparation*, see page 19). This tea has a relaxing effect and it stimulates the appetite.

If the lemon balm tea fails to have the desired effect on you, try a tea blend containing equal parts of lemon balm and hop. The bitter constituents in the hop will stimulate the peptic juice in the stomach, which will increase your appetite (see page 174).

Then eat your supper in peace and quiet and with enjoyment. Eat something light that tastes good to you and agrees with you. Make this meal a festive occasion on a small scale, so that it becomes the crowning event of the day. As soon as you feel tired, go to bed; don't drink coffee to keep yourself awake.

Breakfast is the "medicine" for the entire day. The cardinal rule: Take your time, and eat a variety of foods at breakfast.

Instead of the customary coffee or black tea, try this breakfast tea sometime:

Tea Blend

Chamomile leaves	.70 (20)
Lemon balm leaves	.70 (20)
Peppermint leaves	.35 (10)

Preparation, see page 14.
Application: Drink 8 ounces (1/4 L) of tea in the morning with breakfast.

Try to eat your midday meal in peace and quiet, too—even if the rush of daily activities makes it hard for you.

● **Tea blend**
This tea for nervous stomachs has proved effective in a course of treatment lasting four to six weeks:

Chamomile flowers	1.05 (30)
Lemon balm leaves	.70 (20)
Iceland moss	.70 (20)
Bitter-orange peel	.35 (10)

Preparation, see page 14.

Application: Drink two cups of tea per day, one in the morning and one in the evening.

Flatulence

● **Tea blend**

If gas pains are the primary source of your discomfort, this tea will help you:

Caraway seeds (crushed)	.70 (20)
Peppermint leaves	.35 (10)
Fennel seeds	.35 (10)
Chamomile flowers	.35 (10)

Preparation, see page 14.
Application: Drink up to three cups per day, as needed.

Diarrhea

● **Blueberry decoction**

A blueberry decoction will relieve diarrhea due to a nervous stomach.

Preparation and application: Pour 1 pint (1/2 L) of cold water over 3 heaping teaspoonfuls of dried blueberries, bring to a boil, let simmer over low heat for about 15 minutes. Let the tea cool, then strain and pour it into a bottle. Adults take 1 or 2 tablespoonfuls of it several times (up to ten times) a day; children take 1 or 2 teaspoonfuls each time.

Nausea and Vomiting

● **Tea blend**

For nausea and vomiting in conjunction with a nervous stomach, this tea usually brings swift, sure relief:

Chamomile flowers	.70 (20)
Peppermint leaves	.35 (10)
Lemon balm leaves	.35 (10)
Hop cones	.17 (5)

Preparation, see page 14.

Application: Drink two to three cups per day, as needed.

● **Milk with chamomile tea**

This beverage also has proved efficacious: Mix equal parts of milk and chamomile tea.

Preparation, see page 14.

Application: At bedtime, drink this mixture warm, sipping it slowly.

Lack of Appetite

Children (see page 97) in particular suffer from lack of appetite, but older people and working people can have the same problem. Usually it is caused by some weakness in the digestive tract that can be remedied easily with bitter medicinal teas. The bitter stimulus incites almost all the glands that produce peptic juice to increase their activity, which promotes appetite.

In folk medicine, lack of appetite was seen as the harbinger of various diseases in the digestive tract, as well as a symptom of other, "hidden," illnesses. For this reason people always took it quite seriously and tried to take remedial measures swiftly.

You also should take your lack of appetite seriously and search for the causes. If your lack of appetite persists, a physical examination is essential. If your loss of appetite is the result of a high fever, however, you need do nothing for the time being.

Fever is a defense reaction of the body for which it needs all its "reserves of strength." Eating would place an additional strain on your body. Once the illness has been overcome, your appetite will quickly reappear on its own.

Lack of Appetite in Adults

● **Tea blend**

Often lack of appetite in adults between the ages of twenty and fifty has a mental cause: The stress of daily living is not being handled well—and the stomach and intestines react to this with "weakness." Usually a bitter, aromatic tea blend proves helpful here, and it has a slightly calming effect in addition:

Lemon balm leaves	1.05 (30)
Peppermint leaves	.70 (20)
Wormwood, aerial parts	.35 (10)

Preparation, see page 14.
Application: Drink one cup of tea 30 minutes before meals.

Lack of Appetite in Older People

In old age the activity of all the organs—including the digestive organs—decreases markedly, which frequently results in loss of appetite.

At one time it was believed that the state of health of older people could be improved by a bland diet; consequently, only mild seasonings were used. High-fiber foods, however, were eliminated from the diet altogether; not uncommonly, gruel was the remedy of choice.

Today we know this: The aging organism needs the stimuli provided by highly seasoned foods, so that the glands that produce peptic juice can do their work better. Often the strength of seasonings such as paprika, pepper, or mustard is sufficient to facilitate the conversion of food into substances that the body can use and to stimulate the appetite. Basil, mugwort, marjoram, and summer savory are other recommended seasonings. If you like spicy food, use as much ginger, turmeric, curry, or chili pepper as you like. Attendant symptoms of lack of appetite, such as a feeling of fullness or gas pains after eating, will also improve with proper use of seasonings (see page 113).

● **Tea blend**
A tea with the following composition is highly recommended; it will give you renewed zest for life, help you enjoy your food, and raise your level of vitality:

European centaury, aerial parts	.70 (20)
Bitter-orange peel	.70 (20)

Mugwort, aerial parts	.35 (10)
Yarrow, aerial parts	.35 (10)
Caraway seeds (crushed)	.35 (10)

Preparation, see page 14.
Application: Drink one cup of tea before meals, or three times a day. Granted, this tea has quite a bitter taste, but it is precisely the bitter constituents that make the tea so effective.

Please note
People with allergies should sample this tea blend cautiously at first. There is a danger that itching and inflammatory skin changes will appear in them afterwards (yarrow, mugwort).

● **Tea blend**
This tea has a slightly milder taste and effect:

Hop cones	.35 (10)
European centaury, aerial parts	.35 (10)
Chamomile flowers	.35 (10)
Coriander seeds	.35 (10)
Fennel seeds	.35 (10)
Blackberry leaves	.88 (25)
Raspberry leaves	.88 (25)

Preparation, see page 14.
Application: Drink one to three cups of tea per day, each time before eating.

Diarrhea

With gastrointestinal disorders that manifest themselves as diarrhea, there are clear limits to self-treatment: This symptom may be a sign of serious illnesses.

Please note
If no improvement is seen in cases of diarrhea within two or three days, despite your self-treatment, it is absolutely essential that you place yourself under a doctor's care.

When you suffer from violent bouts of diarrhea, your body loses not only a great deal of fluid, but also the minerals essential for preserving good health. You need to drink plenty of liquids and replace the lost minerals. For this reason, you should add some table salt (about 1/8 teaspoonful per cup is enough) to each cup of tea.

If acute diarrhea comes "like a bolt from the blue," you can assume that it is a defense reaction, triggered by your having eaten something indigestible that your body wants to get rid of quickly. In such cases, severe diarrhea should be looked upon as the body's attempt to cure itself. If vomiting also occurs, it is usually a question of an excessive strain placed on the stomach and intestines by food that is difficult or impossible to digest.

Please note

If there is even the slightest possibility that the severe diarrhea could have been caused by poisoning (mushrooms, plants, chemicals), you must see a doctor immediately!

Indigestibility of Food

● **Charcoal tablets with chamomile tea**
When you need to rule out the possibility that the problems were caused by poisoning, charcoal tablets in combination with a cup of warm chamomile tea (*Preparation*, see page 14) are the proper initial therapy.

Diarrhea Accompanied by Flatulence

● **Erect cinquefoil tea**
You can try to treat diarrhea accompanied by symptoms of fermentation (flatulence and an extremely foul odor) with a medicinal plant that contains tannin. A tea made from erect cinquefoil (*Preparation*, see page 14) will help here.

Application: Drink one to three cups of tea per day, as needed.

● **Tea blend**
This tea also has proved helpful:

Erect cinquefoil, aerial parts	1.05 (30)
Thyme, aerial parts	1.05 (30)
Chamomile flowers	.70 (20)
Peppermint leaves	.35 (10)

Preparation, see page 14.
Application: Drink up to three cups of tea daily.

Constipation

Constipation may be harmless in origin, but it also can be a symptom of serious disease. Therefore, clear limits are set for self-treatment.

Please note

If the constipation has not improved within eight to ten hours after the application of a laxative tea, you must see a doctor.

If the constipation occurs in connection with violent pain in your lower abdomen, go to the doctor at once (suspicion of intestinal obstruction). Under no circumstances should you attempt self-treatment!

Pregnant or nursing women should not drink laxative teas.

Severe Constipation

For the treatment of acute constipation of the bowels, there are many medicinal plants that, when prepared in the form of teas, provide quick relief. These are medicinal plants that contain anthraquinone derivatives as an active ingredient.

● **Tea blend**
I recommend to you a tea made from the leaves or the seedpods of senna and a tea prepared from the bark of alder buckthorn. Try them and decide which agrees with you better:

Preparation: Pour 8 ounces (1/4 L) of boiling water over 1 heaping teaspoonful of senna leaves, senna seedpods, or alder buckthorn bark, let steep for five to ten minutes, and strain.

Application: Drink one cup of tea in the evening before going to bed.

The next morning (it takes six to ten hours to have any effect), a bowel movement will take place. Usually the stool is soft and pasty. If it is watery, cut the dose in half the next time your bowels are constipated.

Please note

Don't let the pleasant effect of these medicinal plants lead you to conclude that you can use them on a continuing basis as a remedy for chronic sluggishness of the bowels. The cause of the chronic constipation has to be treated—go to your doctor.

The continued use of laxatives, even if they are purely herbal in origin, can result in permanent damage—for example, depletion of electrolytes (in particular, loss of calcium), with resulting damage to the heart and circulatory system. Moreover, pigment can be stored in the intestinal mucous membranes and the colon can become irritated.

Chronic Constipation

Important in chronic constipation: Never hold back your stool. At the slightest indication that your bowels want to move, go to the toilet!

● Crushed flaxseed (linseed)

I recommend crushed flaxseed (see page 168) as an effective remedy. The flaxseed swells up in the intestines, which triggers an expansion stimulus that activates peristalsis and thus leads to evacuation; the fat in the flaxseed acts as a lubricant.

Application: Three times a day, take 1 heaping teaspoonful of crushed flaxseed (without soaking it ahead of time) with plenty of water (at least 1 pint [1/2 L]).

● A diet high in roughage, plus exercise

Support this therapy by eating predominantly foods that are high in roughage. Especially recommended are white or red cabbage and high-fiber vegetables like beans, as well as salads made from wild greens, raw vegetables, and high-bulk fruits such as firm apples and pears. In addition, drink plenty of liquids; that is, supply your body with an abundance of fluid. Exercise also plays a major role in regulating your bowel movements. Eat highly seasoned (spicy) foods, as this too makes bowel movements regular.

What should you drink to provide your body with fluids that are not only ample, but also healthful? Neither coffee, black tea, nor soft drinks can serve as healthful thirst quenchers. Coffee and black tea contain caffeine, and soft drinks are high in sugar, which in large quantities is bad for your health.

● Herb tea

I recommend that you drink an herb tea that has a slightly laxative effect due to the fruit acids it contains. It quenches thirst, tastes good, and can be drunk cold, warm, or hot. You can drink this tea at all times, as your "house tea":

Hibiscus flowers	1.05 (30)
Rose hips (with seeds)	1.05 (30)
Raspberry leaves	.35 (10)
Blackberry leaves	.35 (10)
Lemon balm leaves	.17 (5)
Peppermint leaves	.17 (5)

Preparation, see page 14.
Application: Drink up to 1 quart (1 L) of tea per day.

● Tamarind pulp

Finally, I would like to recommend one more old herbal remedy for sluggishness of the bowels that may help you—tamarind pulp. It is available in health food stores.

This substance is the pulp of the fruits of the tamarind tree. It is the fruit acids in this pulp that have a laxative effect (malic acid, succinic acid, citrus acid, and, above all, tartaric acid), and they are supported by invert sugar and potassium bitartrate.

Application: Take 1 tablespoonful of tamarind pulp in the evening, or divide the dose and take 2 teaspoonfuls three times a day. This way your intestines can be "trained to be regular."

● **Prunes and mustard seeds**

Household remedies can be of help also.

Prunes: In the morning, put several prunes in a cup of water to soften; eat the prunes in the evening, and drink the liquid in which they soaked.

White mustard seeds: Three times a day, take 1 teaspoonful of mustard seeds with one cup of water. Both prunes (dried plums) and mustard seeds are available in health food stores.

Gastric and Intestinal Ulcers

The number of people who suffer from gastric or intestinal ulcers grows larger each year. The causes are diverse, but I think that the hustle and bustle of our daily routine has much to do with it. Peace and tranquility and the ability to switch off one's thoughts and relax are therefore important preventive measures. Both types of ulcers, gastric stomach or duodenal, cause pain in the gastrointestinal region and are a great strain on those so afflicted.

Please note

Gastric and duodenal ulcers can be diagnosed and treated only by a physician! The recommendations I offer here are intended only as complementary therapy, to be undertaken only after consultation with your physician.

Gastric and duodenal ulcers may develop when an imbalance arises between the factors that harm the gastric mucosa and those that protect it. The prime necessity, therefore, is to reestablish a state of balance between these factors; only then can the process of healing begin.

Reduction of Excess Gastric Acid

The most important damaging factor is gastric (peptic) acid, and it is crucial to neutralize any excess amount of it or, preferably, to prevent excess production in the first place.

● **Tea blend**

The following tea blend has a slightly calming effect and helps decrease the aftereffects of stress that make people ill. This contributes toward reestablishing the balance between the damaging factors and the protective ones in the stomach. This tea, then, is no typical tea for the stomach and intestines; it can, however, be an effective adjunct to medical therapy.

Lemon balm leaves	1.05 (30)
Valerian root	.35 (10)
Orange flowers	.35 (10)
Fennel seeds	.35 (10)
St. John's wort, aerial parts	.35 (10)
Chamomile flowers	.35 (10)

Preparation, see page 14.

Application: Drink two to five cups of tea per day for a fairly long period (three to four weeks).

● **Cabbage juice treatment**

In clinical tests, a cabbage juice treatment for gastric ulcers also has proved successful. Many patients had no more pain after only a few days, and after several weeks the stomach ulcers were completely healed. The "antiulcer U factor" in cabbage juice stabilizes and strengthens the gastric mucosa.

Application: Drink 1 quart (1 L) of freshly extracted cabbage juice (use a juice extractor) over the course of the day. If flatulence occurs, you can remedy matters by adding 1 tablespoonful of freshly ground caraway seeds.

● **Licorice extract**

The juice extracted from licorice root and licorice root itself have a protective effect on the mucous membranes of the stomach and intestines, as scientific tests have shown. This application, however, absolutely must be discussed with the physician treating you, so that the correct dose for you can be determined.

The standard recipe: Dissolve 1.41 ounces (40 g) of licorice extract in a small amount of water and drink it over the course of the day.

● **Tea blend**

The following tea blend has long proved successful in efforts to soothe the pain of ulcer sufferers. This tea supports both the medical therapy during the acute stage and the follow-up treatment as well:

Chamomile flowers	.88 (25)
Lemon balm leaves	.52 (15)
Iceland moss	.17 (5)
European centaury, aerial parts	.17 (5)
Caraway seeds (crushed)	.17 (5)
(Senna seedpods—only if fairly severe constipation is also present)	.17 (5)

Preparation, see page 14.
Application: Drink two to three cups of tea a day, between meals.

● **Rolling treatment**

The rolling treatment (see page 58) is convincingly successful with gastric and duodenal ulcers, though somewhat time-consuming as well.

● **Proper diet**

In conclusion, a few words about nutrition: Until a few years ago, the diet prescribed for ulcer patients consisted largely of porridge and gruels. Now different rules apply: Everything that agrees with the patient is permitted, including heartily seasoned foods, even those containing paprika or mustard. Bitter foods, however, are to be avoided. I especially recommend that you use cloves as a seasoning, because the essential oil of cloves promotes the healing of gastric ulcers, as scientific research has shown.

Highly seasoned fried foods—in particular, highly seasoned fried onions—often do not agree with ulcer sufferers.

Please note

My statements regarding nutrition where gastric and duodenal ulcers are concerned are not equally binding for all patients. Please discuss the special features of your diet with your physician.

Heartburn, Acid Belching

Acute heartburn after too sumptuous a meal, after misuse of nicotine and alcohol, and, in many people, even after too much coffee, cocoa, or chocolate is usually harmless.

First-aid Measures

I recommend three teas as first-aid measures: chamomile tea; a tea blend containing equal parts of chamomile and lemon balm; and a tea blend consisting of caraway, lemon balm, and chamomile in equal parts.

Preparation, see page 14.
Application: Three times a day, drink one cup of moderately warm tea in sips.

These teas calm the mucous membrane of the stomach. The production of acid is reduced and finally brought back to normal.

Please note

If you frequently suffer from heartburn, it is essential to have your physician identify the cause.

Heartburn at Night

The belching of an acid fluid as the consequence of a weakness in the muscle that constricts the esophagus usually occurs at night and is characterized by the "rising" of partially digested food, mixed with gastric juice, into the esophagus. Little can be accomplished here with medicinal plants. Slightly elevating the upper part of the body in bed has proved helpful. In addition, I recommend that you drink marshmallow tea before going to bed.

● **Marshmallow tea**

Marshmallow tea has to be prepared by the cold-water method, because with this tea it is the dried root that is used as a drug. The root contains, along with the "healing" plant mucilage, a great deal of starch, which in a hot infusion bonds the root cells and prevents the mucilage from finding its way into the tea.

Preparation: Pour 8 ounces (1/4 L) of cold water over 4 heaping teaspoonfuls of marshmallow root, let the mixture stand about two hours or longer, stirring it repeatedly, then strain.

Application: Warm the tea slightly and drink one cup of tea before going to bed. Mixing marshmallow tea with an equal amount of chamomile tea or caraway tea may improve the effect; try it and see what agrees with you best.

Flatulence

This is an extremely troublesome complaint, for which physicians often find no organic cause, even after a thorough examination. Flatulence often is the body's way of expressing emotional disequilibrium and nervousness. Constitutional digestive weakness and digestive processes that have gone awry (for constitutional or emotional reasons) also are possible causes, as is the indigestibility of certain foods, such as legumes and cabbage.

> **Please note**
> Have your physician determine the cause of your flatulence.

Four umbellate plants that make good remedies for flatulence are available to us: caraway, coriander, fennel, and anise. The essential oil they contain has a carminative effect; that is, it causes the release of stomach or intestinal gas.

Indigestibility of Foods

● **Caraway, coriander, fennel, anise**
If you know what dishes you cannot tolerate but would like to continue eating them nonetheless, then you can use these seeds as seasonings, according to taste. Often the culinary dose alone is sufficient to allay the gas pains.

If seasoning does not help, then a tea made from one of these four drugs surely will. Let your taste buds determine which one is right for you; all of them are effective. I attribute the strongest effect to caraway, followed by coriander, fennel, and anise.

Preparation and application: The quantity of the drug needed for the tea depends on the severity of the complaint. Often 1 teaspoonful is enough; sometimes 2 teaspoonfuls are needed. The quantity of tea required is also variable; sometimes just one cup is enough to dispel the gas pains; at other times a second cup of tea is needed after two to three hours. I advise you to experiment: "An ounce of practice is worth a pound of theory."

Crush the seeds (in a mortar) before using them or grind them coarsely (in a spice mill), then pour boiling water over them, let steep for ten minutes, then strain. Drink the tea in sips.

Epigastric Meteorism

Epigastric meteorism is a special kind of flatulence. Gas that collects in the epigastric region presses upward on the diaphragm and constricts the heart, which reacts by causing discomfort.

● **Tea blend**
Quick relief is available in the form of a tea made from caraway and coriander.

Preparation: Mix 1 heaping teaspoonful of caraway with an equal amount of coriander, then crush. Over this mixture pour 8 ounces (1/4 L) of boiling water, let steep in a covered container for about 10 minutes, then strain.

Application: As needed, drink one cup of tea, as warm as possible, in sips.

● **Tea blend**
This tea also has proved reliable for the same purpose:

Chamomile flowers	1.05 (30)
Caraway seeds (crushed)	.70 (20)
Lemon balm leaves	.70 (20)
Coriander seeds (crushed)	.35 (10)
Peppermint leaves	.35 (10)

Preparation and application: As for caraway tea and coriander tea (see page 66).

Please note
It is essential to see a physician if you have heart trouble. The doctor will have to determine the cause.

A Stomach Tea for the Home Medicine Chest

You should keep this tea on hand in your home medicine chest if you have a sensitive, weak, or nervous stomach; your food weighs heavily on your stomach (limited gastric mobility) and you rarely can eat legumes, cabbage dishes, fatty foods, or fried foods without discomfort. You suffer from flatulence and abdominal fullness or lack of appetite. Your nervous stomach also reacts frequently with heartburn and irritations of the gastric mucosa. This tea also helps relieve various digestive complaints. It is suitable for use in a course of treatment, as well as for acute disturbances:

Tea Blend

Chamomile flowers	.70 (20)
Lemon balm leaves	.70 (20)
Peppermint leaves	.70 (20)
Angelica root	.35 (10)
Caraway seeds (crushed)	.52 (15)
Fennel seeds	.35 (10)
Wormwood, aerial parts	.17 (5)

Preparation: Pour one cup of boiling water over 1 heaping teaspoonful of the blend, let steep for three to five minutes, then strain.

Application: As needed, drink one cup of warm tea in sips; alternatively, in a course of treatment, drink two to three cups of tea daily over a period of three to four weeks.

Please note
This tea may not be drunk by anyone with a gastric ulcer!

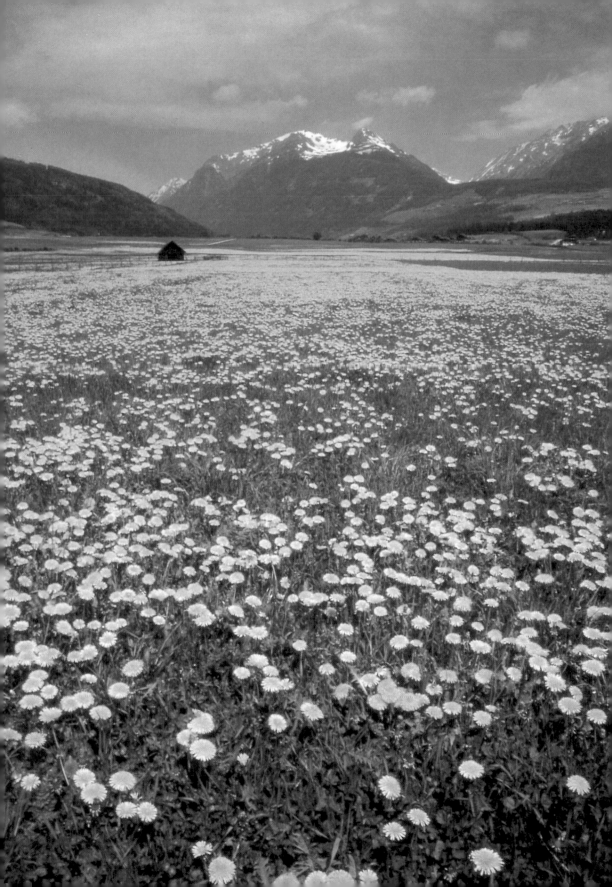

Rheumatism and Gout

← *Dandelion*

What Is Rheumatism— What Is Gout?

Rheumatism and gout are metabolic diseases that can severely impair our general health and that always require medical care. Rheumatism is the name given to flowing twinges of varying intensity in the muscles and joints. The name of this disease comes from the Greek *rheo* = I flow. Rheumatism is a syndrome associated with multiple complaints, of which, as previously stated, pain is the foremost. All the symptoms certainly have different causes. Despite enormous efforts, we still know very little about the causes and the origin of rheumatism. Several factors must combine to trigger this disease, primarily, in all probability, disorders of internal origin that interfere with body metabolism and the workings of the glands and nerves; extraordinary strains (stress); improper diet; lack of exercise; and seats of disease in the body. A hereditary component also may play a role. For this reason, anyone suffering from rheumatism needs to be in a doctor's care. The physician, after detailed examinations, will determine the best possible therapy.

In the case of gout, things are a bit different. Gout is a metabolic disease that is dependent on our diet; it is caused by an excess of uric acid in the blood. Uric acid is formed in the body during the digestion of meat, primarily, and during the catabolism of "used-up" body cells. It normally is excreted through the kidneys along with urine and through the intestines. The production and excretion of uric acid, therefore, are normal metabolic processes. If some imbalance between the production of uric acid and its excretion exists, crystals of uric acid are formed, primarily in the joints. The result is gout, which may also lead to serious systemic diseases. For this reason, the same rule applies to gout: Medical treatment is a prime necessity!

Help from Healing Plants

Medicinal plant applications are appropriate and successful in cases of rheumatism and gout as well, at least as supportive therapy.

I would like to point out emphatically that scarcely any other pathological process is as difficult to influence as chronic rheumatic disease. Although the causes of this disease still are not known precisely, we can assume that they are metabolic disorders of various kinds. Consequently, treatment with medicinal plants is appropriate if it can bring about improvement in the entire metabolic process.

There are a number of medicinal plants that are described by older doctors as antidyscratics. These are medicinal plants that can alter the abnormal "mixture of juices," which is probably what is present in rheumatism. It is quite difficult, however, to undertake a reliable assessment of the action of these plants: First, the form of the complaints varies too greatly from one patient to another; second, the complaints that appear in each patient vary in nature and intensity. Sometimes people feel relatively well, sometimes ill, and sometimes very ill. Thus wrong opinions were formed repeatedly with regard to the efficacy of the medicinal plants that were to be used for treatment. Some were suddenly extolled as miracle cures for no apparent reason and were "in fashion" for a while, only to sink back into oblivion; others were cast aside without reason until they, sometimes only much later, were rehabilitated and joined by new ones. The medicinal plants used to treat gout also experienced ups and downs in the favor of doctors and patients.

In this guide I would like to introduce to you those medicinal plants that really have proved reliable and have been employed by doctors who make intensive use of natural remedies. Among the medicinal plants presented you also will find some whose effect cannot be explained. In folk medicine many of them are considered to be blood purifiers, or depuratives. In fact, it is also important in the treatment of rheumatic disorders and of gout to stimulate the excretory organs—the bladder, kidneys, gallbladder, and liver—and to return sluggish bowel movements to normal regularity. Moreover, through mild healing stimuli, medicinal plants have a positive influence on cell metabolism and on the pathological changes in connective tissue.

Patience Is a Prerequisite

Neither chronic rheumatic diseases nor gout came into being overnight. Wrong directions in body metabolism developed over months, years, often even decades. Anyone who wants to use medicinal plant applications successfully as therapy has to show great patience. In every case, a prolonged course of treatment is required. If you are not willing to use the recommended teas, tea blends, or other applications regularly and over a long period of time, you should not even begin treatment with medicinal plants, because you will meet with failure.

Treatment over time also means that the teas or tea blends employed have to be well tolerated and that, above all, they may not have an unpleasant taste. If possible, they should also have visual appeal. All this I have taken into account and tried to comply with to a large extent. For this reason it is quite important to follow the instructions exactly, even if this should prove somewhat complicated.

Please note

I have already stated clearly that you must discuss with your physician any treatment with medicinal plants. You should never do anything "behind your doctor's back." Side effects and intolerances may come to light, and the efficacy of other medications may be impaired. Your physician is your guide in all cases.

Dandelion—Stinging Nettle—Birch

These three medicinal plants have impressed me favorably because they are convincingly effective. Everyone knows them, everyone can use them as salad greens in spring. Please bear in mind what I have already said: In the use of medicinal plants as supportive treatment for rheumatism and gout, we are concerned in the broadest sense with making a change in body metabolism, stimulating the excretory organs, and employing a mild stimulation therapy.

The leaves and roots of dandelion contain taraxazin, a bitter constituent (which is responsible for the stimulating effect), but additional substances certainly play some role in the action also—enzymatically effective substances, vitamins, trace elements, minerals, and, not least, saponins (see Medicinal Plants and the Substances They Contain, page 8). Most striking is the diuretic effect, which is felt even when a salad of dandelion greens has been eaten.

Because dandelion has long been known as a really good medicinal plant, the list of therapeutic indications is a lengthy one. After careful screening of it, metabolic diseases (such as gout and rheumatism) remain as the area of application. Along with the diuretic effect, mention is made repeatedly of its efficacy in treating gallbladder and liver complaints. The German Office of Health, in the standard permit, makes no mention of its effectiveness in cases of rheumatism and gout, but does acknowledge its metabolism-stimulating, and thus indirectly antidyscratic, properties.

● Hearty Spring Salads

Hearty spring salads are quite effective here. Gather the fresh dandelion leaves, the young stinging nettle leaves (for the sake of expediency, those of the large stinging nettle, *Urtica dioica*), and the birch leaves that are just unfolding. Mince the leaves and add this healthful green seasoning to any clear or thickened soup, vegetable stew, or salad shortly before serving. You also can simply sprinkle the finely chopped leaves onto a piece of buttered bread, mix them with farmer's cheese or another soft cheese, or put them on potatoes. If you do that regularly, you are on your way to stimulating your body metabolism. If these herbs are not aromatic enough for you, you also can use fresh yarrow leaves in spring.

● **Dandelion treatment**

A course of treatment with dandelion tea (dandelion root with the aerial parts) is helpful in treating rheumatic pain of a general nature and, in particular, chronic degenerative joint diseases and gout. For this reason I advise you to use dandelion tea in a course of treatment in spring and fall, because I have repeatedly had news of successes, especially in cases of "joint wear and tear" (arthrosis) and other joint damage (arthritis).

Preparation: Pour 8 ounces (1/4 L) of cold water over 2 heaping teaspoonfuls of the drug (root plus aerial parts), bring slowly to a boil, let steep for 10 to 15 minutes, then strain.

Application: In a course of treatment over a period of at least six weeks (preferably eight weeks), drink two cups of tea per day—after breakfast or with breakfast, and before going to bed.

● **Stinging nettle tea**

The stinging nettle also is an effective metabolic remedy appropriate for application in cases of rheumatism and gout. Recently this medicinal plant became a kind of "fashionable drug"; now stinging nettle tea is being hailed as the remedy of choice for virtually all the troubles of daily life.

I can recommend the use of stinging nettle tea for benign prostate trouble and rheumatic diseases with a clear conscience, because I know the remedy is effective. It is quite helpful in treating gout, in particular, because stinging nettle washes uric acid out of the organism with great force. A course of treatment with stinging nettle tea is also helpful with muscular rheumatism (rheumatoid myositis).

Preparation: Pour 8 ounces (1/4 L) of boiling water over 2 heaping teaspoonfuls of the aerial parts of stinging nettle (the leaves by themselves are preferable, however), let steep for five to ten minutes, then strain.

Application: In a course of treatment lasting three to four weeks, drink three cups of tea per day, between meals.

Please note

After drinking stinging nettle tea, allergies may appear, though rarely. They manifest themselves as edema, skin irritations, urinary retention, or gastric irritations. If allergic symptoms of this kind appear, discontinue treatment with tea immediately. Generally the problems will disappear at once. To be safe, however, you should consult your doctor.

● **Stinging nettle switch**

In any discussion of stinging nettle, it is also necessary to mention the application of the time-tested stinging nettle switch, a practice known as urtication. This treatment, though drastic, is nonetheless effective with sciatica, lumbago, and muscular rheumatism. This application, long forgotten, has been rediscovered. Because some European specialists, including Dr. Rudolf Fritz Weiss, also recommend this application, people once again are putting faith in popular experience and giving urtication a try.

Application of the stinging nettle switch: Whip the painful areas of the body with a switch made of stinging nettle plants tied into a bunch. This procedure has to be carried out on three successive days. Then a break of three days is necessary to prevent sensitization, that is, a long-lasting, overly strong burning sensation on the skin. It is important, Dr. Weiss writes, not to let any cold water touch the treated skin for the rest of the day after urtication has been performed, because the pleasurable feeling of warmth will quickly turn into an unpleasant burning sensation.

● **Birch leaf tea, birch water**

The birch is the third medicinal plant that can be used to ease the pain of people suffering from rheumatism and, above all, from gout, when used for a prolonged period of time. The effect still cannot be explained precisely; we suspect that the substances contained in this medicinal plant have a positive influence on the excretion of uric acid. For medicinal purposes, the parts used are birch leaves

Preparation of birch leaf tea, see page 14.

Application of birch leaf tea: In a course of treatment lasting at least four weeks, drink two to three cups of tea daily, between meals.

The Juniper Berry Treatment

Where juniper berries are concerned, I have a hard time giving the right advice. On the one hand, I am convinced that juniper berries are efficacious; on the other hand, I have to point out the risks of a juniper berry treatment, as the side effects that may appear during it are considerable. Undoubtedly they appear only when an excessively large dose is administered or when the juniper berry treatment is pursued over too long a period of time.

Please note

When there is preexisting damage to the kidneys—for example, if kidney diseases have ever been present at any time—and during pregnancy or for nursing mothers, juniper berries must not be used either in the form of a tea or in the form of a berry treatment!

People with sensitive stomachs should not use juniper berries because of the danger of irritating the mucous membrane of the stomach.

A course of treatment with juniper berry tea (as the German Office of Health states in its recommendations) should never last more than four weeks without consultation with a physician. If the application is continued for a longer term or if the proper dose is exceeded, kidney damage may result, manifesting itself through pain in the kidney region with an increased urge to pass water, painful urination, and the passing of blood and protein in the urine.

Without the approval of your physician, do not take the juniper berry treatment repeatedly recommended in folk medicine. The daily dose increases gradually, reaches a very high level, then decreases again.

The following version of the juniper berry treatment is acceptable, and it also is advised by doctors of naturopathy. It should be performed twice a year, each time for a period of 24 days. Thus its duration is within the limits of the four-week application period approved by the German Office of Health.

Application: The first day, take four berries—all of them at once or over the course of the day (at the beginning of the treatment, either way is possible). From the second day on, take one more berry each day than you did the previous day, until the daily dose totals 15 berries. The more berries you take each day, the more important it is to distribute them over the course of the day. I consider it advisable to divide the berries into three or four daily doses, drinking at least one full glass of water with each dose. Once you have reached a daily total of 15 berries, reduce the amount by one berry per day until you finally reach the initial dose of four berries again.

Elderberry Flowers and Linden Flowers

In folk medicine, these two medicinal plants have a firm place. In Europe, many legends and superstitions are centered around these trees. In Germany the elderberry bush was considered the abode of Mother Hulda, the protectress of house and home. Linden wood was used for carving sacred works of art, and the linden tree, which was the village tree, played an important role in the life of early Europeans. Thus it is only natural that special curative power was ascribed to these two medicinal plants. Much of it is certainly exaggerated, but both elderberry flowers and linden flowers can be recommended, either singly or in tea blends, as mild sudorifics and metabolic stimulants in the treatment of rheumatism and gout.

Preparation of both teas: Both linden flower tea and elderberry flower tea are prepared as infusions. Pour 8 ounces (1/4 L) of boiling water over 2 teaspoonfuls of the drug, let steep for ten minutes, then strain.

This method of preparation is applicable also for rheumatism teas, which contain other medicinal plants along with these two drugs.

Application: In a course of treatment lasting three to four weeks, drink two to three cups of tea per day—to prevent profuse sweating, drink the tea slowly, moderately warm, and in sips.

Other Medicinal Plants as Remedies for Rheumatism and Gout

In searching for additional medicinal plants to use as rheumatism teas, I tracked down several that have proved reliable in tea blends or as single teas.

Goutweed (*Aegopodium podagraria*), a common garden weed, when drunk as a tea eases the pain of gout. Used as salad greens, it should also play an important role in the diet of gout patients.

Pansy (*Viola tricolor*) and eyebright (*Euphrasia officinalis*) are also classed with the antidyscratics, that is, those medicinal plants that can effect a positive change in the abnormal "mixture of juices." Both these medicinal plants are used to treat rheumatism and gout, primarily in tea blends, along with sea sedge (*Carex arenaria*), bean hulls (*Phaseoli vulgaris*), chickweed (*Stellaria media*), herb mercury (*Mercurialis annua*), goldenrod (*Solidago virgaurea*), or common field horsetail (*Equisetum arvense*).

Easing Rheumatic Pain

● **Tea treatment**
Two other medicinal plants, willow (*Salix*) and meadowsweet (*Filipendula*)—both contain salicylic compounds—are also helpful in easing rheumatic pain in many cases. They should be drunk as a tea in a course of treatment.

Preparation of willow bark tea and meadowsweet tea, see page 14.

Application of both teas: In a course of treatment lasting three to four weeks, drink two to three cups of tea per day. After one week, stop for two to three days, then resume the tea treatment.

● **Tea blends**
Unfortunately, none of the many useful medicinal herbs is able to cure chronic rheumatism. It is also impossible to stipulate which of them should be given preference in therapeutic use. For this reason, tea blends generally are used in treating rheumatism.

The following rheumatism tea blends have been put to the test many times and are drunk by many people afflicted with rheumatism. You will have to try them out and see which blend agrees with you and/or which blend helps you.

Tea Blend 1	oz. (g)
Elderberry flowers	.35 (10)
Common or field horsetail, aerial parts	.35 (10)
Stinging nettle leaves	.35 (10)
Dandelion roots (with aerial parts)	.35 (10)
Birch leaves	.35 (10)

Tea Blend 2	
Willow bark	.35 (10)
Birch leaves	.35 (10)
Linden flowers	.35 (10)
Eyebright, aerial parts	.35 (10)
Pansy, aerial parts	.35 (10)
Dandelion roots (with aerial parts)	.35 (10)

Tea Blend 3	
Bur (burdock) roots	.35 (10)
Meadowsweet, aerial parts	.35 (10)
Sea sedge rhizome	.35 (10)
Bean hulls	.35 (10)

Tea Blend 4	
Goldenrod, aerial parts	.35 (10)
Birch leaves	.35 (10)
Willow bark	.35 (10)
Common or field horsetail aerial parts	.35 (10)
Meadowsweet, aerial parts	.35 (10)
Elderberry flowers	.35 (10)

Tea Blend 5

Elderberry flowers	.35 (10)
Juniper berries (crushed)	.35 (10)
Stinging nettle leaves	.35 (10)
Birch leaves	.35 (10)
Dandelion roots (with aerial parts)	.35 (10)

Preparation of these tea blends: Pour 8 ounces (1/4 L) of cold water over 2 heaping teaspoonfuls of the blend in question, bring slowly to a boil, let steep for five minutes, then strain.

Application of these tea blends: In a course of treatment lasting four to six weeks, drink two to three cups of tea per day.

Please note
If, contrary to expectation, gastrointestinal upsets occur, discontinue the treatment at once. You may then try a different tea blend. Talk to your doctor beforehand.

Stimulating the Excretion of Uric Acid

● **Tea blends**
The following tea blends have proved helpful in treating gout, by stimulating the excretion of uric acid and easing pain, and also as a dietary food:

Tea Blend 1

Goutweed leaves	.35 (10)
Elderberry flowers	.35 (10)
Linden flowers	.35 (10)
Dandelion roots (with aerial parts)	.35 (10)

Tea Blend 2

Sloe or blackthorn flowers	.35 (10)
Pansy, aerial parts	.35 (10)
Elderberry flowers	.35 (10)
European alder-buckthorn bark	.17 (5)

Tea Blend 3

Rhubarb roots	.35 (10)
Senna seedpods	.35 (10)
Elderberry flowers	.35 (10)
Peppermint leaves	.17 (5)
Rose hips	.17 (5)

Preparation of these tea blends: Pour 8 ounces (1/4 L) of boiling water over 2 level teaspoonfuls of the blend in question, let steep for five to ten minutes, then strain.

Application of these tea blends: In a course of treatment lasting four weeks, drink two to three cups of tea daily.

Please note
Tea blends 2 and 3 contain medicinal plants with a laxative effect. If this effect is too powerful and the stool is watery rather than pasty, discontinue the treatment.

Indigestion

● **Tea blends**
Teas for gout patients with impaired liver function, that is, with indigestion (inability to digest fat) or constipation:

Tea Blend 1

Dandelion roots (with aerial parts)	.70 (20)
European centaury, aerial parts	.35 (10)
Milk thistle fruits (crushed)	.35 (10)
Peppermint leaves	.35 (10)
Celandine roots	.17 (5)

Tea Blend 2

Peppermint leaves	.35 (10)
Dandelion roots (with aerial parts)	.35 (10)
Wormwood, aerial parts	.17 (5)
Lovage roots	.17 (5)
Raspberry leaves	1.05 (30)

Preparation of these tea blends: Pour 8 ounces (1/4 L) of boiling water over 1 to 2 heaping teaspoonfuls of the blend in question, let steep for five minutes, then strain.

Application of these tea blends: In a course of treatment lasting three to four weeks, drink two to three cups of tea daily.

A Rheumatism and Gout Tea for Your Home Medicine Chest

It is not to everyone's liking to search for a suitable tea by lengthy experimentation, although I strongly advise that you do so, because—particularly with rheumatism and gout—scarcely any tea is equally effective for all people. There is, however, one tea blend that I often have recommended with success:

Stinging nettle leaves	.88 (25)
Dandelion roots (with aerial parts)	.88 (25)
Birch leaves	.52 (15)
Raspberry leaves	.52 (15)
Willow bark	.35 (10)
Hibiscus flowers	.35 (10)

Preparation, see page 14.

Application: In a course of treatment lasting at least three weeks, drink two to three cups of tea daily.

Can Rheumatism and Gout Be Prevented?

Gout, I believe, can certainly be prevented, because it is a "disease of affluence," which occurs particularly when too fatty, too ample, or too unbalanced a diet is eaten. This is not the place to present a detailed diet for gout sufferers, but I would like to give you a few rules to follow in deciding what to eat. Because brains, kidneys, sardines packed in oil, chocolate, cauliflower, asparagus, and meat promote gout on the basis of the substances they contain (purines), you should exclude these foods from your diet. Spinach, legumes, peaches, grapes, and apricots also should be avoided. Alcohol often triggers the first attack of gout.

People afflicted with gout have to be careful all their lives not to eat anything that promotes the production of uric acid and has a negative influence on its excretion. Help in choosing the right foods is available in nutritional guides and food tables, which you will find listed on page 224, under Books for Further Reading.

Time-tested Home Remedies

How can you prevent gout or rheumatic disorders with the aid of medicinal plants? Here I can only offer what is employed time and time again in folk medicine. I cannot vouch for the efficacy of the home remedies recommended. These applications, however, are found in all the older books of home remedies, and they surely are present there because they have been identified as helpful. Here are a few samples:

● **Pressed juice of rowanberries**
The juice extracted from rowanberries (the berries of the European mountain ash, or rowan, *Sorbus aucuparia*) mixed with honey is held to be a preventive for rheumatism. In a course of treatment lasting four to six weeks, drink 4 ounces (1/8 L) of freshly pressed, boiled rowan-

berry juice mixed with 1 tablespoonful of honey, apportioned over the course of the day.

Cider vinegar with honey

Cider vinegar with honey is also recommended. Mix 4 ounces (1/8 L) of water with 1 teaspoonful of cider vinegar and 1 teaspoonful of honey, and drink this mixture before breakfast.

Pointer: Diabetics should not apply these two home remedies, because they contain honey.

European cowslip root tea

The tea made from European cowslip roots (*P. veris*) is also considered a preventive for rheumatic pain, to be used by people who have a family history of rheumatism, that is, people in whom a hereditary component can be anticipated.

Preparation: Pour 8 ounces (1/4 L) of boiling water over 2 level teaspoonfuls of chopped European cowslip roots, let steep for 15 minutes, then strain. Primrose (*P. vulgaris*) roots may be used here as well.

Application: Twice a year, in a course of treatment lasting three to six weeks, drink one to two cups of tea daily, as warm as possible.

> **Please note**
>
> Because European cowslip roots contain a great many saponins, gastrointestinal irritations are possible. If stomach pain, nausea, or diarrhea occurs, discontinue the treatment.

Herbal Baths

With rheumatism and gout, more than with almost any other maladies, baths have an impressive record of easing pain. Experience has taught us this. I recommend, above all, baths using hayseed, rosemary, horsetail, or marsh tea (Labrador tea) and, for the sake of experiment, also baths with juniper berries, lavender, or yarrow.

Preparation of the recommended baths for rheumatism; the quantities given are sufficient for one full bath:

Hayseed bath

Pour 5 quarts (5 L) of water over 10.58 to 17.63 ounces (300–500 g) of hayseed, bring to a boil, let boil for about 15 minutes, then strain. Add the extract to the bath water.

Temperature of bath water, 95 to 100.4°F (35–38°C), length of bath, 15 minutes. Rest after bathing.

Rosemary bath

Pour 1 quart (1 L) of water over 1.76 to 2.11 ounces (50–60 g) of rosemary leaves, bring slowly to a boil, let steep for 10 to 15 minutes, then strain. Add the extract to the bath water.

Temperature of bath water, 95 to 100.4°F (35–38°C), length of bath, 10 to 15 minutes. Rest after bathing.

Horsetail bath

Soak 3.52 ounces (100 g) of horsetail (aerial parts) in 2 quarts (2 L) of hot water for about one hour, then bring the mixture briefly to a boil and strain. Add the extract to the bath water.

Temperature of bath water, 98.6 to 100.4°F (37–38°C), length of bath, 15 minutes. Rest after bathing.

Marsh tea bath

Pour 3 quarts (3 L) of boiling water over 3.52 ounces (100 g) of marsh tea leaves, let steep for half an hour, then strain. Add the extract to the bath water.

Temperature of bath water, 98.6°F (37°C), length of bath, 10 to 15 minutes. Rest after bathing.

Juniper berry bath

Pour 3 quarts (3 L) of boiling water over 3.52 ounces (100 g) of crushed juniper berries, let steep for half an hour, then strain. Add the extract to the bath water.

Temperature of bath water, 100.4°F (38°C), length of bath, 10 minutes. Rest after bathing.

Lavender bath

Pour 1 quart (1 L) of water over 1.76 to 2.11 ounces (50–60 g) of lavender flowers, bring to a boil, let steep for ten minutes, then strain. Add the extract to the bath water.

Temperature of bath water, 96.8 to 100.4°F (36–38°C), length of bath, 15 minutes. Rest after bathing.

● **Yarrow bath**
Pour 2 quarts (2 L) of water over 7.05 ounces (200 g) of yarrow (aerial parts), let boil for ten minutes, then strain. Add the extract to the bath water.

Temperature of bath water, 98.6°F (37°C), length of bath, 15 minutes. Rest after bathing.

You may be able to buy ready-made extracts in some health food stores. Please follow the instructions for use included in the package.

> **Please note**
> Medicinal baths may place a strain on your heart and circulatory system. Please ask your physician whether he or she advises the use of these baths.

Hayseed Poultice

Hot hayseed or flaxseed poultices have also proved useful in cases of rheumatism, particularly muscular rheumatism, for their ability to stimulate circulation and thus to ease pain. Please follow the directions carefully; this application has optimum effect only when performed correctly.

Preparation, see page 46.

Application: The hayseed or flaxseed poultice should remain in place for 20 minutes, unless it has cooled to such an extent that warmth can no longer be felt.

Embrocations

People afflicted with rheumatism and gout use liniments and salves (embrocations) just as much as baths, because they improve the mobility of the muscles and joints. The pain is eased as well. Of the commercially available salves, oils, and lotions made from medicinal plants, I recommend the oil of St. John's wort for use as a liniment with muscular rheumatism and as a soothing poultice with gout. I also recommend arnica ointment and calendula ointment. Other ointments, or salves, made from plant resins or essential oils can also help people suffering from rheumatism and gout. It is scarcely advisable to make these salves yourself, as top-quality products are available in pharmacies and health food stores.

I also would like to give mention to three liquid embrocations that once were quite popular for their power to stimulate the circulation and to allay pain, but then fell into obscurity: spirit of camphor, spirit of ants (formic acid), and spirit of mustard. The latter two are difficult to find, but spirit of camphor is available in some pharmacies. Please follow directions on the label for use.

Rheumatism Teas

About 25 years ago, a medicinal plant from Africa appeared on the market in Germany and attracted great attention because it, as is often the case, was extolled as a miracle drug for arthrosis (wear and tear of the joints) and arthritis (inflammations in the joints, articular rheumatism). The "miraculous" element was emphasized even more by the high price demanded for it. This plant is African devil's claw (*Harpagophytum procumbens*), a member of the Pedaliaceae family (see page 139). The storage roots of this visually striking plant yield the tea drug, devil's claw, *Harpagophyti radix* (*Radix* or *Tubera Harpagophyti*).

Unfortunately this African devil's claw, as it more accurately should be called, is frequently confused with another "devil's claw" of the species *Phyteuma*.

● **Devil's claw tea**
Although the devil's claw (also called rampion) that grows in northern latitudes is not used for medicinal purposes, the devil's claw tea made from the African devil's claw has indeed proved

valuable in treating rheumatic complaints, in particular, chronic arthritis.

Preparation: Pour 10 ounces (300 mL) of boiling water over 1 heaping teaspoonful of finely chopped devil's claw root and set aside for six to eight hours. Stir the tea mixture occasionally. After straining, bring the tea briefly to a boil again, then let it cool to drinking temperature. Because the tea should be apportioned over the course of the day, I recommend that it be put while still hot into a thermos jug, to be poured as needed.

Application: In a course of treatment lasting three to six weeks, drink 8 ounces (1/4 L) of moderately warm tea, distributed over the course of the day.

Please don't expect too much of this tea; it is no wonder drug. Because there are few workable remedies for rheumatic pain, however, it does expand the available selection of effective medicinal plants. In any event, it is worth a try.

In addition to its soothing effect on rheumatism sufferers, devil's claw tea reputedly also has a positive effect on gastric, intestinal, gallbladder, and liver ailments, which is common to almost all bitter drugs. It is also said that the tea can lower elevated levels of cholesterol and blood lipids.

● **Tea blends that contain bitter constituents**

In conjunction with the research done on the African devil's claw, whose bitter constituents are viewed as active substances, this question arose: Can an antirheumatic effect be imputed to all medicinal plants with bitter constituents? The question has not yet been answered satisfactorily, but more and more people are voicing the opinion that there is a connection between bitter constituents in medicinal plants and effectiveness against rheumatism.

I offer this tea blend of bitter or bitter and aromatic drugs for you to sample:

Tea Blend 1

Gentian root	.70 (20)
European centaury, aerial parts	.70 (20)
Mugwort, aerial parts	.35 (10)
Bitter-orange peel	.35 (10)

Preparation: Pour 8 ounces (1/4 L) of lukewarm water over 2 level teaspoonfuls of this blend, let steep about half an hour, then strain.

Application: In a course of treatment lasting at least three weeks, drink two to three cups of tea daily.

If the taste of this tea is too bitter for you, you can correct it slightly by adding medicinal plants with fruit acids. Appropriate additions are hibiscus flowers and rose hips.

Tea Blend 2

Gentian roots	.70 (20)
European centaury, aerial parts	.70 (20)
Mugwort, aerial parts	.35 (10)
Bitter-orange peel	.35 (10)
Iceland moss	.35 (10)
Hibiscus flowers	.35 (10)
Rose hips (with seeds)	.35 (10)

Preparation: Pour 8 ounces (1/4 L) of boiling water over 2 heaping teaspoonfuls of this blend, let steep for five to ten minutes, then strain.

Application: In a course of treatment lasting three to four weeks, drink two to three cups of tea daily.

I would also like to acquaint you with a time-tested recipe to combat rheumatism taken from an old pharmacy journal. It was written down about 120 years ago.

Tea Blend 3

Lovage roots	1.76 (50)
Angelica roots	1.76 (50)
Willow bark	3.52 (100)
Peppermint leaves	3.52 (100)
Black currant leaves	3.52 (100)
Elderberry flowers	7.05 (200)
European alder-buckthorn bark	3.52 (100)

Preparation, see page 14.
Application: Drink two cups of tea daily.

Please note

At one time every rheumatism tea had to contain a laxative drug, in this case, alder buckthorn bark. I find it preferable to replace this ingredient with 3.52 ounces (100 g) of rose hips with seeds. This does not change any of the instructions for preparation and application.

Blood-purifying Treatments

"Blood-purifying" treatments, which continue to enjoy universal popularity, are usually carried out in spring or, more recently, also in fall. Their purpose is to mobilize the body's powers of resistance. With the help of these treatments, rheumatism and gout can be prevented and rheumatic complaints can be alleviated.

In spring, the emphasis is on stimulating excretion. For this reason, tea blends and plant juices are employed to stimulate the activity of the kidneys. Medicinal plant preparations that are considered to be liver stimulants are used, as are, frequently, laxatives—usually in the form of senna leaf tea, senna seedpod (mother-leaf) tea, rhubarb root tea, or alder buckthorn bark tea.

No objection can be made to "blood purification," except to the extended use of the laxative teas, which leads to electrolyte depletion. "Blood purification" really does create a new sense of well-being, particularly in conjunction with a reduction in the amount of food you eat.

As for plant juices and extracts, preference should be given to dandelion, stinging nettle, horsetail, and birch-leaf. Most tea blends intended as spring tonics contain stinging nettles, birch leaves, and dandelion roots (with the aerial parts). The aerial parts of goldenrod, pansies, horsetail, and eyebright; elderberry flowers; linden flowers; fennel seeds; chamomile flowers; and rose hips are also frequently used as single teas or in tea blends. A great many of these medicinal plants are also contained in rheumatism teas or in bladder and kidney teas—precisely because a metabolic effect is being aimed at. In addition to these ingredients, drugs that have a pleasant aroma or an attractive appearance also have a role to play, for spring teas need to look appetizing as well as to smell good.

The following tea blends have proved helpful, particularly for rheumatism and gout patients.

● **Herbal breakfast tea**

A tasty herbal breakfast tea without any laxative drugs:

Birch leaves	.35 (10)
Fennel seeds (crushed)	.35 (10)
Rose hips (with seeds)	.35 (10)
Hibiscus flowers	.35 (10)
Chamomile flowers	.35 (10)
Linden flowers	.35 (10)
Dandelion roots (with aerial parts)	.35 (10)
Lemon balm leaves	.35 (10)
Peppermint leaves	.35 (10)
Pansies, aerial parts	.35 (10)

Preparation: Pour 8 ounces (1/4 L) of boiling water over 2 heaping teaspoonfuls of this blend, let steep for about five minutes, then strain. Because fairly large quantities usually are needed, I recommend that you go ahead and prepare this tea by the quart. For 1 quart (1 L) of water you will need 3 tablespoonfuls of this tea blend.

Application: In a course of treatment lasting four to six weeks, drink three cups of tea daily.

● **Tea blends**

A tea for rheumatism and gout patients who suffer from sluggishness of the bowels:

Tea Blend 1

European alder-buckthorn bark	.35 (10)
Fennel seeds (crushed)	.35 (10)
Goldenrod, aerial parts	.35 (10)
Hibiscus flowers	.35 (10)
Chamomile flowers	.35 (10)
Peppermint leaves	.35 (10)
Pansies, aerial parts	.35 (10)
European centaury, aerial parts	.35 (10)
Stinging nettle leaves	.17 (5)
Senna leaves	.17 (5)
Pot marigold flowers	.17 (5)
Sandalwood (red)	.17 (5)

Preparation: Pour 8 ounces (1/4 L) of boiling water over 2 heaping teaspoonfuls of this blend, let steep for three to five minutes, then strain. Sweetening with honey is recommended (diabetics do not sweeten).

Application: As needed, drink two cups of tea daily.

Pointer: Alder buckthorn bark and senna leaves, contained in tea blend 1, are fairly powerful laxatives. Although only moderately high doses of them are present in the following blend, the stool may nonetheless become too soft. If this happens, discontinue the treatment. Then you can choose either the first or the third blend.

A tea for reducing or fasting, intended especially for overweight people with rheumatism or gout:

Tea Blend 2

Maté leaves (green)	1.05 (30)
Hibiscus flowers	.70 (20)
Rose hips (with seeds)	.35 (10)
European alder-buckthorn bark	.17 (5)
Birch leaves	.35 (10)
Stinging nettle leaves	.35 (10)
Dandelion roots (with aerial parts)	.35 (10)

Preparation: Pour 8 ounces (1/4 L) of boiling water over 2 heaping teaspoonfuls of this blend, let steep for five to ten minutes, then strain.

Application: In a course of treatment lasting four to six weeks, drink two to three cups of tea daily.

A tea for removal of water, especially in cases of gout:

Tea Blend 3

Stinging nettle leaves	.35 (10)
Birch leaves	.35 (10)
Goldenrod, aerial parts	.35 (10)
Dandelion roots (with aerial parts)	.35 (10)
Horsetail, aerial parts	.35 (10)
Rose hips (with seeds)	.35 (10)
Peppermint leaves	.35 (10)

Preparation and application of this tea blend, as for tea blend 2.

Pointer: Accumulations of water in the body that are due to poor performance of the heart or kidneys should not be treated with this tea without consultation with your physician!

Here is a tea for use as a spring and fall tonic by people who want to stimulate their powers of resistance because they catch cold in every draft, get flulike infections several times a year, and have trouble recovering from illnesses. This tea is also recommended for use in "blood purification" by people with rheumatism and gout.

Tea Blend 4

Linden flowers	.70 (20)
Elderberry flowers	.70 (20)
Iceland moss	.70 (20)
Chamomile flowers	.70 (20)
Fennel seeds (crushed)	.35 (10)
Rose hips (without seeds)	.35 (10)
Eyebright, aerial parts	.35 (10)
Bitter-orange peel	.35 (10)
Hibiscus flowers	.17 (5)
Pot marigold flowers	.17 (5)
Lavender flowers	.17 (5)

Preparation and application of this tea, as for tea blend 3.

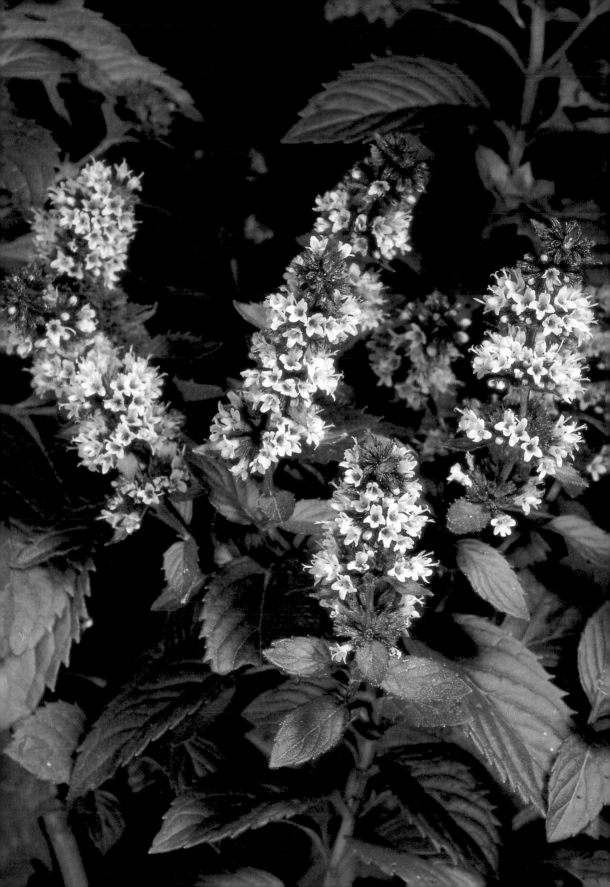

Gallbladder and Liver Complaints

← *Peppermint*

Medicinal Plants That Act on the Gallbladder and Liver

The most significant problems caused by the gallbladder are usually painful, because gallstones, disturbances in bile discharge, and inflammations of the gallbladder and bile ducts are involved. The pain, of course, then brings the sufferers to the doctor at once; this is quite important, as successful treatment can begin only after an exact diagnosis.

The doctor's efforts can be supported quite well with medicinal plants, and you also can try to allay or cure less serious cases with self-medication. There are a great many medicinal plants worth recommending here. My favorites are peppermint leaves, yarrow (aerial parts), dandelion roots with the aerial parts, celandine leaves, fumitory (aerial parts), stinging nettles (aerial parts), and the umbellates anise, fennel, caraway, and coriander. Chamomile, lemon balm, European centaury, and wormwood are also of great value, of course.

Please note

The treatment of liver diseases with teas made from medicinal plants is somewhat more difficult. For this reason, I strongly advise that even the slightest suggestion of liver disease serve as an inducement for an immediate visit to your doctor. The following symptoms must be taken very seriously:
● Tenderness in the liver region caused by enlargement of the liver.
● Yellowing of the skin or of the white of the eye.
● White coloration of the stool and coffee-brown urine.

Itching, redness of the palms, and fatigue in combination with indigestion also may indicate the presence of liver disease. With symptoms of this kind, a doctor must be consulted at once!

Symptoms and Their Treatment

Gallstones

If the doctor discovers gallstones in your X ray, he or she will usually suggest that they be surgically removed. Gallstones are unpredictable in that they may be "quiet" for years, then trigger severe colics that block the common bile ducts, which results in further damage.

If surgery is not possible or if the patient rejects it, the question naturally arises whether there is not some tea that, if drunk as a precautionary measure, can prevent gallstone colic. And in fact, the bitter or bitter and aromatic medicinal plants have proved useful as preventives.

Troublesome Gallstones

● **Wormwood tea, European centaury tea**
People who suffer from gallstones usually know in advance that a colic attack is on its way. If they then drink hot wormwood tea (*Preparation*, see page 14) in sips, the gallstone will become quiet again; the dreaded colic attack will not occur. Centaury tea (*Preparation*, see page 14) can be expected to have a similar effect.

● **Tea blends**
Two tea blends that I consider especially effective with a troublesome gallstone have the following composition:

Tea Blend 1

To quiet the gallstone:	oz. (g)
Wormwood, aerial parts	.70 (20)
Peppermint leaves	.35 (10)
Chamomile flowers	.35 (10)

Tea Blend 2

Antispasmodic tea for patients with gallstones:	
Celandine roots	.35 (10)
Wormwood, aerial parts	.35 (10)

Caraway seeds (crushed)	.35 (10)
Peppermint leaves	.35 (10)
Lemon balm leaves	.35 (10)
Fumitory, aerial parts	.35 (10)

Preparation of these tea blends, see page 14.

Application of these tea blends: In a severe case, drink one cup of tea, unsweetened, very warm, and in sips. With persistent cramplike pain and until the doctor clarifies the situation, drink one cup of tea three times daily.

Preventing the Formation of Stones

Anyone who has been freed of gallstones through surgery would naturally like to know how to counteract the renewed formation of gallstones.

● **Tea treatment with dandelion**
It has become apparent that a course of tea treatment that includes dandelion can prevent the new formation, as well as the enlargement, of gallstones (of kidney stones too, incidentally; see page 72). This has been adequately proved on the basis of experience, although the operative mechanism thus far has not been studied in detail.

The hope tied to this—of dissolving existing gallstones with a dandelion treatment—has not become a reality.

> #### Please note
> Dandelion should not be used with inflammation or blockage of the common bile ducts! It is important that in undertaking a dandelion tea treatment, which you should do only after consultation with your physician, you adhere conscientiously to the guidelines.

Preparation: Pour 1 quart (1 L) of cold water over 8 heaping teaspoonfuls of dandelion roots with the aerial parts (available in pharmacies), bring to a boil and allow to boil for one minute; take the decoction off the heat, let it steep for five minutes, then strain. Pour the tea into a thermos bottle.

Application: Drink the dandelion tea in sips during the course of the day—unsweetened, please! If 1 quart (1 L) of dandelion tea is too much liquid for you, you may drink somewhat less. This treatment should be carried out in spring and in fall over a period of six to eight weeks.

Pointer: People with rheumatism, especially those who suffer from chronic articular rheumatism, will find this tea treatment equally beneficial (see page 72).

● **Tea blend**
A tea blend for stone prevention, also useful as protective liver therapy and as a metabolic stimulant:

Milk thistle fruits (crushed)	1.05 (30)
Dandelion roots (with aerial parts)	.70 (20)
Stinging nettle leaves	.70 (20)
Birch leaves	.35 (10)

Preparation, see page 14.

Application: As for dandelion tea (see page 72). This tea blend may be drunk in alternation with dandelion tea; it is advisable to alternate every other day.

● **Oil of St. John's wort**
Oil of St. John's wort, according to folk medicine, stimulates bile production and cures bile flow disorders. It may be difficult to find in North America.

Application: Take 2 to 3 teaspoonfuls of oil daily.

● **Turnip and turnip juice**
In folk medicine, both applications are considered well-established preventives for gallbladder trouble.

I am reluctant to pass on recommendations from folk medicine that are hard to explain, but this is an exception. Statistics show that in areas where many turnips are eaten (the large white turnips eaten with beer) fewer gallstone operations are necessary. During the periods when fresh turnips are available, try to eat them daily, for example, as a salad, with bread and butter, or with cheese. If you dislike turnips, you can also drink the commercially available turnip juice (or prepare it by using a juicer): 1 tablespoonful three times a day. In any event, it is good for you.

Preventing Liver Complaints

Milk thistle fruits rank in first place here. The active complex they contain, silymarin, protects the liver and has a regenerative effect on the fatty liver so common today; that is, it renews the cells. Dandelion stimulates the activity of the liver cells, and peppermint leaves also are reputed to be "liver-friendly." Hepatitis—which urgently requires medical attention—often leaves behind serious permanent damage if the patient does not strictly avoid everything that harms the weakened liver. Alcohol, for example, is truly forbidden until lab tests over a lengthy period of time show normal results once more. Usually a special diet or certain bland foods are prescribed for people with liver trouble. Anyone who wishes to speed recovery by drinking liver teas should talk this over with his or her physician.

● **Tea blends**
I recommend the following tea blends, in which dandelion and milk thistle complement one another admirably in their effect.

Tea Blend 1

Dandelion roots (with aerial parts)	.35 (10)
Milk thistle fruits (crushed)	.70 (20)

Tea Blend 2
Peppermint used as a third medicinal plant will increase bile flow in addition:

Milk thistle fruits (crushed)	.70 (20)
Dandelion roots (with aerial parts)	.35 (10)
Peppermint leaves	.35 (10)

Tea Blend 3
Especially well suited for abdominal fullness after meals:

Milk thistle fruits (crushed)	.52 (15)
Dandelion roots (with aerial parts)	.52 (15)
Peppermint leaves	.52 (15)
Caraway seeds (crushed)	.17 (5)

Preparation, see page 14.
Application: In a fairly lengthy course of treatment—four to six weeks, for example—drink one cup of tea daily.

Inflammations of the Gallbladder or Bile Ducts

The following tea blends are eminently suitable as adjuncts to medical procedures.

Feeling of Pressure, Burning Pain

● **Tea blend**
Counteracts an annoying feeling of pressure in the area of the gallbladder and a moderately severe pain that is experienced as a burning sensation, usually accompanied by loss of appetite:

European centaury, aerial parts	.35 (10)
Peppermint leaves	.35 (10)
Yarrow flowers	.35 (10)
Chamomile flowers	.35 (10)

Flatulence

● **Tea blend**
For gas pains after meals:

Chamomile flowers	.35 (10)
Peppermint leaves	.35 (10)
Caraway seeds (crushed)	.35 (10)
Fennel seeds (crushed)	.35 (10)
Coriander seeds (whole)	.17 (5)

Cramplike Pain

● **Tea blend**

Relieves cramplike pain:

Chamomile flowers	.35 (10)
Peppermint leaves	.35 (10)
Lemon balm leaves	.35 (10)
Celandine roots	.35 (10)
Fumitory, aerial parts	.35 (10)
Caraway seeds (crushed)	.35 (10)

Pain after Eating

● **Tea blend**

Relieves or eases pain, feeling of pressure, and flatulence that occur regularly after eating. A decrease in the emptying out of bile must be assumed:

Peppermint leaves	.70 (20)
Stinging nettle leaves	.70 (20)
Chamomile flowers	.70 (20)
Coriander seeds (whole)	.35 (10)

Sluggishness of the Bowels

● **Tea blend**

Cures sluggishness of the bowels in gallbladder complaints of various kinds:

Senna leaves	.35 (10)
Senna seedpods	.35 (10)
European alder-buckthorn bark	.35 (10)
Lemon balm leaves	.35 (10)
St. John's wort, aerial parts	.35 (10)
Fennel seeds (crushed)	.35 (10)
Anise seeds (crushed)	.35 (10)
Caraway seeds (crushed)	.35 (10)
Wormwood, aerial parts	.35 (10)
European centaury, aerial parts	.35 (10)

Preparation of all tea blends, see page 14.

Application of all tea blends: Drink either one cup of tea in the evening as needed, or two to three cups of tea daily after eating, on a regular basis. None of the tea blends recommended may be drunk longer than three weeks in a row. After an interval of several weeks, the three-week tea treatment may be repeated.

Please note

If no long-lasting improvement has occurred, it is essential to consult a doctor once more.

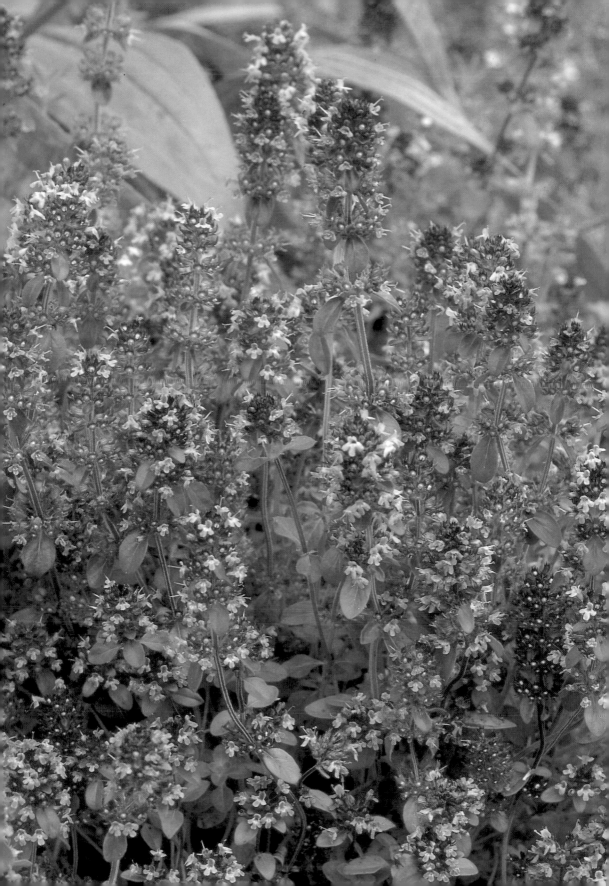

Childhood Diseases

← *Thyme*

Complaints of Infants and Young Children

Most of the complaints from which infants and young children suffer may, in terms of their nature, resemble the complaints that trouble adults. Children are not small adults, however; even medicinal plant applications, which often can be used to ease their discomfort, have to be specially prepared and administered in the proper dose. Sometimes these complaints are indispositions typically found in infants and small children, which require special treatment.

> **Please note**
> I am assuming that you have provided your child with the recommended medical checkups. I am also taking it for granted that you immediately seek medical advice for your child in the event of any unclear findings, high fever, or severe pain. Self-help with Healing Plants (see page 5) should not tempt you to want to cure everything yourself. With children's complaints as well, medicinal plant therapy has its limits. Please pay careful attention to the general advice on The Limits of Self-treatment (see page 7) and the special pointers in this chapter.

Gas Pains, Nutritional Disorders

Breast-fed babies generally have little trouble with the intake and digestion of their nourishment. If the mother, in addition, eats properly during the breast-feeding phase—if, for example, she eliminates from her diet all foods that cause flatulence and avoids substances such as alcohol, coffee, and black tea—she generally can be almost certain that her baby will not have to suffer from lack of proper nutrition.

● **Fennel tea**
Babies that are bottle-fed rather than breast-fed, however, quite often are plagued with gas pains

or a feeling of fullness after eating, and the consequences usually are restlessness, fretfulness, or screaming. Sometimes just changing the formula (powdered milk) is sufficient.

If switching to a different formula doesn't help either, however, and if the gas pains persist, then catnip and fennel elixir is worth a try. You can buy catnip and fennel elixir in some pharmacies; follow the label directions.

● **Homeopathic remedies**
In especially stubborn cases, above all when your baby cannot get any rest, homeopathy has also proved helpful. I recommend *Chamomilla* 6x: Three times a day, give the baby five pellets with the formula in the bottle. It is also available in drop form; follow the label directions. First, however, please discuss this application with your pediatrician.

● **Marjoram ointment**
A mild salve containing marjoram can also help alleviate gas pains in infants: Gently rub the ointment into the area around the baby's navel. You can make marjoram ointment yourself.

Preparation: Pour 1 teaspoonful of vodka or some other pure grain alcohol (i.e., *undenatured ethyl alcohol*; CAUTION: **not rubbing alcohol!**) over 1 teaspoonful of powdered marjoram and let the mixture stand for several hours. Add 1 teaspoonful of fresh, unsalted butter and warm the mixture over hot water for about ten minutes. Then strain through a handkerchief or a small piece of gauze and allow to cool.

Diarrhea and Restlessness During the Teething Phase

Diarrhea during teething, also called "teething diarrhea," is a frequent occurrence in infants. Although we are told that teething itself cannot cause diarrhea—teething is not a disease, but a natural process—experience teaches us that the two often coincide, perhaps because the young child's resistance is lower at this time, perhaps also because rubbing the itching gums with the hands or with unclean objects (toys) enables germs and/or zymogens (proenzymes) to reach the stomach and intestine.

● **Blueberry tea**

Here rapid improvement can be brought about with a tea made from dried blueberries.

Preparation: Pour 1 pint (1/2 L) of cold water over 3 heaping teaspoonfuls of dried blueberries, bring to a boil, and allow to boil down for about 15 minutes. Let the tea cool, strain it through a cloth, then filter it through a coffee filter.

Application: With your doctor's approval, add 1/2 to 1 teaspoonful of this tea to the formula in the little patient's bottle three to five times a day.

Usually the diarrhea will disappear after two days at most. If that is not the case, the doctor has to be consulted again.

● **Chamomile tea**

Children over one year old can also be given 1 ounce (30 ml) of chamomile tea (*Preparation*, see page 14) per day, mixed with 1 teaspoonful of blueberry tea, in their bottle of formula.

> **Please note**
> Diarrhea in infants and young children is by no means harmless. At any rate, the doctor should find out the cause.

● **Homeopathic remedies**

Teething children frequently suffer not only from diarrhea, but also from agonizing restlessness at the same time. They want to be carried around all the time and scream at once when they are put down to sleep.

Chamomile in a homeopathic preparation is helpful here. Every hour, put 1 or 2 drops of *Chamomilla* 4x directly in the mouth of your little patient, who will quickly lose his or her restlessness and sleep well.

Colds in Infants

A cold is quite unpleasant, especially in infants and young children, because the swollen mucous membranes in the nose make breathing through the nose difficult or even impossible. Eating can suddenly become a problem for both bottle-fed and breast-fed babies. Their sleep is disturbed as well, and the general health of the little children deteriorates noticeably. For this reason, help is necessary. There are drops that will reduce the swelling of the mucous membranes, but pediatricians do not like to prescribe them.

● **"Inhalations" with chamomile tea**

Chamomile is extremely beneficial in such cases. For this purpose, prepare an infusion with chamomile flowers and place it in a bowl next to the bed.

Preparation and application: Pour 1 pint (1/2 L) of boiling water over 5 tablespoonfuls of chamomile flowers and let steep, covered, for ten minutes. Pour this infusion, while still hot, into a bowl and set it next to the child's bed or crib. The chamomile vapors, which are breathed in as with an inhalation, cause the swelling in the nasal mucous membranes to subside. Often improvement is seen even overnight. It has also proved helpful to hang cloths soaked in chamomile tea on a line in the child's room.

● **Marjoram ointment**

To ease the discomfort, I also recommend marjoram ointment, which you can make yourself (*Preparation*, see page 90). Spread a little of it on the bridge of the nose or under the nose on the upper lip of the little patient. Mothers who have tried this gentle treatment are full of praise for it.

> **Please note**
> With high fever or if the little patients have an earache—which they make known by rubbing their ear with their fist—a doctor should be consulted without delay.

Coughs

● **Marshmallow syrup**

A simple cough, which younger children get frequently, can best be treated with the time-tested marshmallow syrup, which you can make yourself.

Marshmallow Syrup (15 portions)   *oz. (g)*
Coarsely chopped marshmallow
   root   .07 (2)
Pure grain alcohol*   .03 (1)
Water   1.58 (45)
Sugar   2.22 (63)

Preparation: Pour the grain alcohol* and the water over the marshmallow root, placed on a filter, and let steep for one hour at room temperature, repeatedly pouring back over the filter the liquid that has dripped down. Over low heat, dissolve the 2.22 ounces (63 g) of sugar in 1.30 ounces (37 g) of the liquid thus obtained, and bring it briefly to a boil. Let the finished syrup cool and transfer it to a small bottle (keep in the refrigerator).

The amounts given may of course be doubled or multiplied further in order to make more syrup.

Application: Administer 1 teaspoonful of syrup three to five times a day, spread over the course of the day.

Important: Marshmallow syrup is not suitable for children with diabetes!

● **Tea blends**

This tea blend has also proved a reliable remedy for coughs in young children from one to five years of age.

Tea Blend 1
Thyme, aerial parts   1.05 (30)
Fennel seeds (crushed)   .70 (20)
English plantain leaves   .70 (20)
Mullein flowers   .35 (10)
High mallow leaves   .35 (10)
Lemon balm leaves   .35 (10)

Preparation, see page 14.
Application: Drink one cup of tea several times a day.

For a dry cough, which usually appears at the start of a cold, administer this tea:

Tea Blend 2
High mallow flowers   .70 (20)
Mullein flowers   .17 (5)
Fennel seeds   .17 (5)
Anise seeds   .17 (5)

Preparation: Pour 8 ounces (1/4 L) of water over 2 teaspoonfuls of this mixture, bring to a boil, let steep for five minutes, then strain.
Application: Drink one cup of tea two to three times daily, sweetened with honey or sugar (for diabetics, without honey or sugar).

Whooping Cough

This infectious disease, a typical childhood disease, must by all means be treated by a physician. Your doctor, however, usually will be quite appreciative of well-tried aids from the realm of botanical medicine.

● **Thyme tea**
One medicinal herb has proved especially reliable in treating whooping cough: thyme. Its antispasmodic properties ease the whooping cough and reduce the number of coughing fits. Only the doctor can decide whether the little patients can be given thyme tea (*Preparation*, see page 14), and if so, how much. This decision will depend on the child's age.

● **"Inhalations" with thyme tea**
Using thyme tea as an "inhalant" is also helpful. To do so, prepare a tea, then pour the hot infusion into a bowl and place it beside the child's bed. This hot thyme infusion, applied in the form of vapor, is suitable for both infants and young children.
Preparation and application: As for chamomile vapor, see page 14.

---

*For example, vodka or some other *undenatured ethyl alcohol*; CAUTION: **do not use rubbing alcohol!**

● **Thyme bath**

In addition, thyme baths, which have an anti-spasmodic effect, also have proved helpful with young patients (from the first year on).

Preparation, see page 39.

Application: The little patient should take a thyme bath approximately every other day. The temperature of the bath water should be 98.6°F (37°C); the length of the bath, ten minutes.

● **Tea blend**

Also reliable as a remedy for spasmodic coughs and whooping cough in young children (from one to five years of age) is the following tea blend—but please consult the pediatrician in charge before you administer it.

European cowslip roots	.35 (10)
English plantain leaves	.35 (10)
Thyme, aerial parts	.35 (10)
Burnet roots	.17 (5)
Iceland moss	.17 (5)
Fennel seeds	.17 (5)

Preparation: Pour 8 ounces (1/4 L) of water over 2 teaspoonfuls of the mixture, bring to a boil, let steep for five minutes, then strain.

Application: Drink one cup of tea two to three times daily, sweetened with honey or sugar (for diabetics, unsweetened).

● **Homeopathic remedies**

Here too I would like to recommend two herbal homeopathic remedies that are quite effective in the initial stages of colds and coughs, above all, whooping coughs. *Aconitum* 4x (made from monkshood, or aconite) is helpful in treating colds accompanied by fever that were caused by drafts and cold wind; administer two to three drops of it five to eight times daily. *Drosera* 4x (made from sundew, or drosera) helps ease dry, barking coughs (abdominal whooping cough); administer two drops of it every hour. In place of the drops, you also can use pellets (one drop = one pellet), as they are prepared without alcohol.

Measles, Chicken Pox, Mumps

The dangerous childhood diseases, such as measles, chicken pox, and mumps, also have to be treated by a doctor, of course, like all colds accompanied by fever.

● **Tea blend**

To support the measures taken by the doctor, however, the following tea blend is especially well suited, because it fosters recovery and is drunk willingly by feverish children. (Discuss this with the doctor.)

Rose hips (with seeds)	1.05 (30)
Linden flowers	.35 (10)
Lemon balm leaves	.35 (10)
Chamomile flowers	.35 (10)

Preparation: Pour 8 ounces (1/4 L) of boiling water over 2 teaspoonfuls of this mixture, let steep for 15 minutes, then strain and sweeten with honey (for diabetics, no sweetening).

Application: Several times a day, give the patient one cup of lukewarm tea to sip—to quench thirst as well.

Asthma

Asthma is a malady affecting children that is becoming increasingly common. Its causes are allergic in part. If breathing becomes difficult and labored, and wheezing noises are heard as the child inhales, immediate medical examination and treatment are required.

● **Tea blend**

The following tea blend is an excellent adjunct to your doctor's therapy. It has become apparent that if this tea is applied, the asthma attacks not only become less frequent, but also take a less severe course.

Elderberry flowers	.70 (20)
High mallow flowers	.52 (15)
Fennel seeds	.17 (5)

Preparation: Pour 8 ounces (1/4 L) of hot water over 1 heaping teaspoonful of this mixture, let steep for ten minutes, then strain and sweeten with 1 teaspoonful of honey (for diabetics, no sweetening).

Application: Drink one cup of tea in the morning and another in the evening.

● **Homeopathic remedies**

Here the homeopathic preparation made from elderberry *(Sambucus nigra)* also has proved reliable. It brings perceptible relief. *Sambucus nigra* 3x: Put 20 drops in half a glass of water; during the asthma attack have the little patient drink a small swallow every 10 to 15 minutes.

> **Please note**
> Every self-medication has to be discussed with the pediatrician in charge.

Sleep Disturbances

When infants and young children will not or cannot sleep, they usually are troubled by pain. As a rule the causes are digestive upsets such as gas pains or pain in the stomach. Often the cause may also be a slight head cold that makes breathing through the nose difficult, or it may be the gums that itch and burn when the teeth are breaking through. (Remedies for these complaints are found on pages 90 and 91.) If the applications presented there do not result in success, then a trip to the doctor is unavoidable. Only a physician can identify and treat the cause.

● **Homeopathic remedies**

Among young children, even among infants, there are some real squallers—I describe them as homeopathic "*Chamomilla* types"—little tyrants who are perpetually in a foul mood if they are not being carried around. As soon as you put them down again, the bawling starts anew. Teething is especially problematic for these children, and fever, earache, and foul-smelling diarrhea are quite common in them. Of course it is advisable to ask the doctor, but expe-riences teaches that serious diseases rarely lie at the root of these problems.

The homeopathic remedy *Chamomilla* 6x will help here: Dissolve five to ten pellets in some water and have the child drink it five times a day. (Drops may be used in the same manner as the pellets.)

Bed-wetting

Children who have completed their third year are usually able to control the release of their urine. They are "dry," as mothers put it. If a child in the fourth year of life is still wetting the bed at night, some pathological disorder is generally present.

> **Please note**
> Because this disorder has a great many possible causes, it is absolutely essential to have a doctor examine the child!
> If the doctor finds that organic diseases or abnormalities are present in the kidney and bladder area, the malady can be treated resolutely and usually successfully as well. If, however, some general developmental delay is the cause, it is best to be patient a while longer; the disorder may disappear without having to be treated.

Most children who are still wetting the bed after their third birthday, however, are disturbed in their emotional development and in many cases need the help of a child psychologist or psychotherapist. Parents need to know that neither rebukes nor threats nor punishment are likely to be successful measures; even restricting a child's intake of fluids or getting him or her up at night will only cause harm.

Sympathy and understanding are the best way to help your child, who needs to be aware of your love at all times! Give your child affection, loving attention, and plenty of time for cuddling. Telling stories and reading aloud are often the best medicine to make this emotional disturbance disappear.

In such cases, teas and other preparations made from medicinal plants can support your own efforts.

● St. John's wort tea

St. John's wort has proved highly reliable, particularly in a fairly lengthy course of treatment with tea.

Preparation: Pour one cup of boiling water over 1 heaping teaspoonful of St. John's wort (aerial parts), let steep for five to ten minutes, then strain.

Application: In the morning and at noon, administer one small cup of St. John's wort tea; it may be sweetened with honey (for diabetics, no sweetening). If the little patient is allowed to put the honey in the tea himself or herself, this medicine works even better!

● Tea blend

The following tea blend is also recommended:

St. John's wort, aerial parts	.70 (20)
Lemon balm leaves	.35 (10)
Orange flowers	.17 (5)

Preparation and application, as for St. John's wort tea. This tea also can be sweetened with honey, unless the child is diabetic.

● Tea blend

With pediatric patients (three years of age and up), the tea made from the aerial parts of the passionflower plant has proved reliable as a mild sedative and tranquilizer. I recommend its application as a complementary therapy for bed-wetting in children. It is most effective in a blend with St. John's wort and a tonic (strengthening) medicinal plant, perhaps centaury or bitter-orange peel.

Passionflower, aerial parts	.70 (20)
St. John's wort, aerial parts	.52 (15)
Bitter-orange peel	.35 (10)
European centaury, aerial parts	.17 (5)

Preparation and application, as for St. John's wort tea.

● Small aids

The following two methods of combatting bedwetting may also serve as small aids drawn from empirical medicine:

It has become apparent that massaging the inner thighs with the oil of St. John's wort increases the sensitivity of the bladder sphincter and thus is effective with nighttime bed-wetting.

In addition, it has been observed that many children wet the bed only when they sleep on their back. If you can get them used to turning onto their side to sleep, this can be quite helpful. (The child automatically will turn onto his or her side if you can tie a knot in the diaper [or other garment] at the rear, at the child's back).

● Homeopathic remedies

Plantago 3x, a medicament made from greater plantain—which is quite common in this country—has proved reliable as a homeopathic remedy:

Administer 3 to 5 drops twice a day.

Avena, the homeopathic original tincture made from oats, is rightly recommended in books of home remedies: In the evening take ten drops with some sugar (diabetics should put the drops in water).

Complaints of Children and Adolescents

With the complaints of older children and adolescents (five to fourteen years of age), too, the symptoms often resemble those that appear in adults. Here as well the treatment has to be determined by the patient's age.

Stomachache, Vomiting

These complaints are common in children, as well as in adolescents, who, for example, have trouble resisting the ice cream and cake served at children's birthday parties or on other festive occasions.

Nausea and even vomiting (a defense reaction of the overloaded stomach) are the consequences of indiscriminate "gorging." Often cramplike pain, termed "bellyache" or "tummyache" by children, also appears. Similar complaints occur when the stomach is "shocked" by overly cold drinks (straight from the refrigerator).

● **Chamomile or peppermint tea**
A cup of chamomile tea or peppermint tea (*Preparation*, see page 14), drunk as warm as possible and in sips, usually brings instant relief. In any event, you should give your child a second cup to drink after one hour has passed and a third cup shortly before bedtime. The tea will soothe the irritated gastric mucous membrane, halt inflammations, and ease tension.

> **Please note**
> Nausea, vomiting, and "tummyache" may also be initial symptoms of a serious illness, such as appendicitis! Get the doctor involved at once, if the complaints have not completely vanished within a few hours of drinking the recommended tea.

Diarrhea or Constipation

In general, children and adolescents very rarely suffer from chronic diarrhea or chronic constipation. If one or the other does occur, have the doctor identify the cause so that it can be treated.

● **Chamomile tea**
Severe diarrhea, however, is a common digestive disturbance at this age, though it usually does not last long. Often chamomile tea can help here to set things right again.
Preparation, see page 14.
Application: Drink one or two cups of tea when the trouble appears.

● **Tea blend**
This tea is also a time-tested source of immediate relief:

Chamomile flowers	.70 (20)
Erect cinquefoil roots (tormentil)	.88 (25)
Peppermint leaves	.35 (10)

Preparation, see page 14.
Application: As needed, drink one to three cups daily.

● **Tea blend**
For severe constipation, which also occurs from time to time in children and adolescents, I recommend the following tea:

Senna leaves	.70 (20)
Chamomile flowers	.35 (10)
Peppermint leaves	.35 (10)
Caraway seeds (crushed)	.35 (10)

Preparation, see page 14.
Application: As needed, drink one cup of tea. If no bowel movement has occurred after eight hours, drink one more cup of tea.

> **Please note**
> If that still has no effect, you need to consult a doctor.

Lack of Appetite in Children

Many things can cause a loss of appetite in children: eating sweets between meals, drinking too many sweet soft drinks, and feeling worry and anxiety as well (search for the cause!). If these factors can be ruled out, then digestive weakness is present; the stomach and intestines do not react with sufficient vigor after food is eaten.

Two medicinal plants offer themselves for use in treating a lack of appetite due to digestive weakness: European centaury and bitter-orange peel. European centaury is a pure bitter-constituent plant, whereas the peel of bitter oranges tastes bitter and aromatic at the same time. The bitter constituents stimulate the glands that produce peptic juice, which in turn stimulates the appetite.

● **Tea blends**

A tea prepared from equal parts of the aerial parts of European centaury and bitter-orange peel will quickly help you regain a healthy appetite.

Preparation, see page 14.

Application: Usually it is sufficient to give children several tablespoonfuls of this tea before meals and immediately thereafter. Do not sweeten it under any circumstances!

This tea blend has also proved to be a good remedy for lack of appetite:

Tea Blend

Bitter-orange peel	.70 (20)
Rose hips (with seeds)	.70 (20)
Peppermint leaves	.35 (10)
Wormwood, aerial parts	.17 (5)

Preparation, see page 14.

Application: Drink one cup of tea half an hour before meals.

● **Lingonberry jam**

Lingonberry jam, which you can buy in some grocery stores and some gourmet shops, has an aperitive effect. Give your child 1 teaspoonful of lingonberry jam three times a day.

You will observe that your child enjoys eating this jam as long as his or her lack of appetite caused by digestive weakness persists. Once the digestive weakness has been remedied and a healthy appetite has been restored, the child will no longer want to eat the jam. Do not force him or her to do so, as this rejection is a healthy reaction that tells you that the digestive weakness has been overcome.

● **Sloe jam**

Sloe jam also can stimulate a child's appetite. This is especially true of children who are not "morning people" and are unable to eat breakfast. Give your child 1 teaspoonful of sloe jam before he or she gets out of bed. Then the child is hardly apt to reject breakfast; moreover, he or she will have renewed interest in eating.

Lack of Appetite in Adolescents

The same recommendations that I made for children apply also to adolescents (ages ten to twenty) who suffer from a lack of appetite due to digestive weakness.

If adolescents "lose their appetite" because they are suffering from emotional stress, then the recipes that I recommend for lack of appetite in adults between twenty and fifty years old are suitable (see page 60).

School Problems, Examination Phobia, Restlessness

Quite often even children and adolescents are no longer able to cope with everyday stress: Excessive demands made upon them in school, noise disturbance, and exposure to continuous stimuli are the most common causes. The symptoms are feelings of reluctance, loss of volition, irritability, nervousness, and sleep disturbances. If these children are not helped, a general fear of life and organic diseases such as stomach ulcers may develop.

Please note

In every case of this kind you should seek the advice of an experienced physician. Under no circumstances should you take it upon yourself to give your child tranquilizers—not even if they are promoted as mild and harmless. Pills do not solve any problems!

You as parents are first challenged to take steps when you notice that your son or daughter feels out of sorts. At the very least, you should try to talk to your child about his or her problems when the report card states that lack of concentration, decline in performance, and loss of volition are the reasons for the bad grades. On no account should you punish your child!

Better organization of work, more appropriate use of free time, elimination of outside stimuli—to the extent possible—and sometimes a change of school as well can remedy the situation. The advice of an experienced educator or psychologist may be quite valuable in deciding how to best help your child.

Here I would like to tell you how you can help your child with preparations made from medicinal plants. Because children and adolescents usually react quite well to mild phytotherapeutic drugs (remedies derived from medicinal plants), you can achieve quite a lot on your own.

Sleep Disturbances, Nervousness

● **Passionflower tea**

The aerial parts of the passionflower plant have proved especially useful in pediatric practice. A tea is helpful with patients who experience difficulty going to sleep, anxieties, restlessness, and general nervousness.

Preparation, see page 14.

Application: In a course of treatment lasting four to eight weeks, drink one or two cups of tea daily and one additional cup before going to bed.

Passion fruit juice has a relaxing and calming effect and is available in health food stores.

Drinking 3.52 ounces (100 g) of it over the course of the day will help to calm your child.

● **Lemon balm tea**

I also recommend lemon balm as a medicinal plant for use in treating sleep disturbances and nervousness in children. A tea made from lemon balm leaves will be especially helpful if the child has trouble assimilating the impressions and demands of the past day.

Preparation, see page 19.

Application: Drink one cup of tea in the evening.

● **Chamomile tea**

Chamomile is also highly effective in children and adolescents. Give the patient chamomile tea with milk and honey (for diabetics, unsweetened).

Preparation and application, see page 14.

Nervousness and Aggression

● **Tea blend**

With general nervousness and aggressiveness, this tea has proved especially reliable as a house beverage, to be served at breakfast and with the evening meal.

Lemon balm leaves	.70 (20)
Passionflower, aerial parts	.70 (20)
Chamomile flowers	.70 (20)
St. John's wort, aerial parts	.70 (20)
Blackberry leaves	.70 (20)
Raspberry leaves	.35 (10)
Hibiscus flowers	.35 (10)
Rose hips (with seeds)	.35 (10)

Preparation: Pour 1 pint (1/2 L) of boiling water over 2 tablespoonfuls of this blend, let steep for five minutes, then strain. The tea may be diluted with lemon, or thinned with milk and sweetened with honey (for diabetics, no sweetening).

Lack of Appetite, Loss of Volition

● **Tea blend**

If lack of volition and poor performance are accompanied by lack of appetite, then I recommend—also as a house beverage—this tea:

Lemon balm leaves	.70 (20)
Passionflower, aerial parts	.70 (20)
Blackberry leaves	.70 (20)
European centaury, aerial parts	.17 (5)
Orange flowers	.17 (5)

Preparation, see page 14.
Application: Drink two to three cups of tea daily.

Upset Stomach

● **Tea blend**

If excessive demands and stress have "upset the stomach" of your son or your daughter, this tea will help:

Chamomile flowers	1.05 (30)
Lemon balm leaves	.70 (20)
Iceland moss	.70 (20)
Hibiscus flowers	.35 (10)

Preparation: Pour 8 ounces (1/4 L) of boiling water over 2 teaspoonfuls of this blend, let steep for five minutes, then strain.
Application: In the evening drink one cup of unsweetened tea, as warm as possible, in sips.

Loss of Appetite Accompanied by Flatulence, Feeling of Fullness

● **Tea blend**

With loss of appetite that is accompanied by a feeling of abdominal fullness or by flatulence, caused by nervousness and excessive demands (school stress), this is the remedy of choice:

European centaury, aerial parts	.17 (5)
Hop cones	.17 (5)
Lemon balm leaves	.35 (10)
Iceland moss	.35 (10)
Strawberry leaves	.35 (10)

Preparation, see page 14.
Application: Drink one small cup of tea about 20 minutes before each main meal.

Restlessness

● **Mixture of tinctures**
These drops, which you can mix yourself, have proved reliable as a general tranquilizer, especially for children and adolescents.

Tincture of valerian	.35 (10)
Tincture of oats (homeopathic original tincture)	.35 (10)
Tincture of passionflower plant (homeopathic original tincture)	.35 (10)

Application: Depending on the patient's age, take 5 to 10 (up to 20) drops with sugar (diabetics should use water) three times a day.

Colds

Illnesses caused by colds, including coughs, head colds with paranasal sinusitis, sore throat, and tonsillitis, are usually triggered by viruses. They are best countered by preventive measures: herbal teas, inhalations, or gargling with disinfectant herbs (see Colds, page 30).

On pages 91 and 92 you will find special recommendations for complaints of this kind in infancy and early childhood; for older children and adolescents, however, the recommendations given for adults are applicable.

Acne

In treating this skin disease, which afflicts primarily adolescents of either sex, it is advisable to fall back repeatedly upon the experience of folk medicine. Hyperactivity of the sebaceous glands results in comedos, or "blackheads and whiteheads," pimples, and pustules that clog the pores of the skin. Blackheads are sebaceous plugs in the pores that have turned black through contact with the air, in contrast to whiteheads, which are cut off from the air by a thin layer of skin. Pimples and pustules are comedos that have become inflamed. Left untreated, they may leave unsightly scars after they heal.

Eruptions of acne are not contagious, as acne is based on a change in certain bodily functions during puberty. Many adolescents are so badly afflicted that acne represents an emotional problem for them, as well as a "cosmetic problem."

The teas recommended for treating acne cannot cure the disease, of course, but they certainly assist the healing process. Used regularly, these teas will at least make the course of this skin disease less severe.

● **Pansy or violet tea**
The wild pansy (violet) ranks in first place, in my opinion.

Preparation, see page 14.

Application: In a course of treatment lasting six to eight weeks, drink two to three cups per day; in addition, dab lukewarm to warm tea (whatever is tolerable) on the affected areas of skin daily.

● **Tea blends**
Pansy tea also can be mixed with a like amount of chamomile tea. Iceland moss and couch grass root round out the medicinal plant therapy; they can be used both internally, as a tea, and externally, as a facial wash. I recommend the following tea blends:

Tea Blend 1
As a wash:

Pansies, aerial parts	.70 (20)
Iceland moss	.35 (10)
Couch grass roots	.35 (10)

Tea Blend 2
As a wash and a drink:

Chamomile flowers	.35 (10)
Iceland moss	.35 (10)
Eyebright, aerial parts	.35 (10)
Pansies, aerial parts	.35 (10)

Tea Blend 3
As a drink:

Couch grass roots	.35 (10)
Pansies, aerial parts	.35 (10)
Horsetail, aerial parts	.35 (10)
Stinging nettle leaves	.35 (10)
Dandelion roots (with aerial parts)	.35 (10)

Preparation of these tea blends: Pour 8 ounces (1/4 L) of lukewarm water over 2 heaping teaspoonfuls of the blend in question, let steep for three to five hours, stirring frequently, then strain.

For the application, the tea is warmed: for drinking, to normal drinking temperature; for use as a wash, to about 104°F (40°C). If you are afraid of transferring germs to the diseased skin along with the tea (a fear I think is groundless), the tea can be heated briefly to the boiling point after it is strained.

Internal application: Drink two to three cups of tea daily. A course of treatment lasting six to eight weeks is advisable twice a year.

External application: Dab the tea infusion on the affected areas daily; choose whatever temperature—lukewarm to warm—is tolerable.

● **Homeopathic remedies**
With acne it is also worth trying two homeopathic remedies, *Viola odorata* 3x and *Arctium lappa* 3x. *Viola* is the sweet-smelling violet, from which this homeopathic medicine is made; *Arctium* is burdock. Take these two remedies in alternation, for example, *Viola odorata* 3x in the morning and *Arctium lappa* 3x in the evening; the first three days take 5 drops three times per day, thereafter 3 drops three times per day.

Handy Pointers

● With warts, massage with castor oil several times a day is sometimes helpful. This remedy is said to be especially successful with large warts.

● With low blood pressure, from which growing children sometimes suffer, a cold shower every morning is helpful. First shower at the usual temperature, then finish with a cold shower lasting only a few seconds. Bathing the fore arms with cold water from time to time is also thought to raise blood pressure slightly.

● With freckles, slices of cucumber are said to be helpful. Lay them on the affected areas.

● With school stress, passion fruit juice can be of use one glass twice a day; young girls are helped by relaxing lavender baths.

● Two homeopathic remedies, *Avena sativa* (oats) in the original tincture and *Chamomilla* at the fourth or sixth decimal potency (4x or 6x), are often beneficial. Mix equal parts of these two remedies, and take 5 to 10 drops twice a day.

● With watering eyes, which many children get in the slightest draft, a mixture of equal parts of fennel tea and eyebright tea (*Preparation*, see page 14) can help. Drink one cup of tea three times a day.

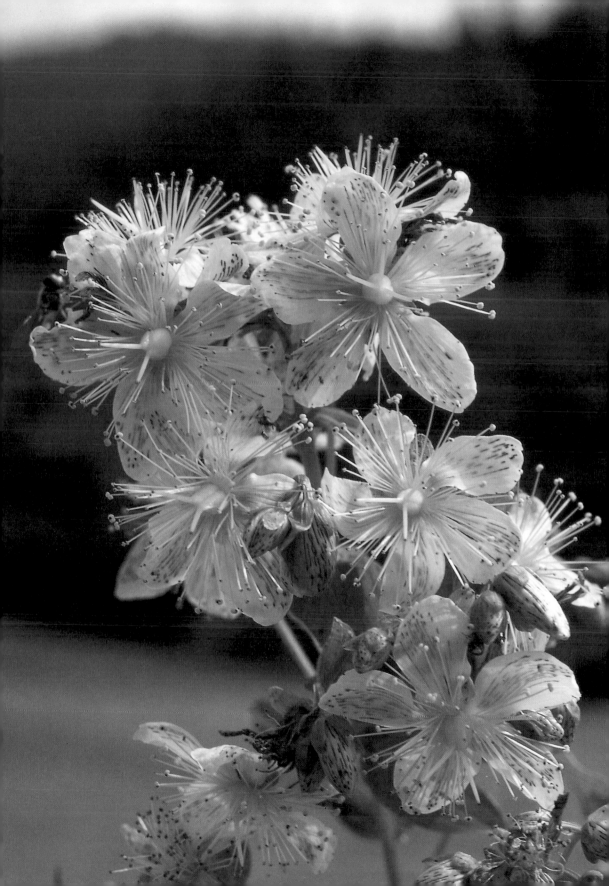

Gynecological Complaints and Menopause

← *St. John's Wort*

Gynecological Complaints

It may be more accurate to speak of indispositions, rather than of complaints, that women and girls have to endure. Gynecological complaints in the sense of organic diseases, of course, need to be treated by a physician. Because the numerous, supposedly innocuous complaints may be early signs of serious diseases, however, before treating yourself with healing plants you should make certain that the problems really are only minor indispositions. These may include menstrual complaints; nervous upsets; inactivity; mild premenstrual depression; constitutional leukorrhea; neurodystonia of the true pelvis, accompanied by problems such as lower back pain, twinges in the breasts; premenstrual colic pain; and the various complaints of menopause as well.

To treat these complaints I can offer medicinal herbs, which—with your doctor's approval— are suitable as adjunct therapy. In mild cases, they also can be called upon for use in self-treatment.

Menstrual Complaints

In connection with a woman's monthly cycle, complaints of different kinds often appear. The most common symptoms are these: before, during, and after menstruation, twinges, aches, or cramps in the lower abdominal region, usually in various locations, connected with pain in the breasts and lower back; occasionally also feelings of nausea, headaches, or migraines.

Twinges, Aches

● **Three teas**
Menstrual pain in young girls often is severe and relatively long-lasting. Especially at the onset of the menstrual period, the pain usually is experienced as severe.

Ideally before the first menstrual period and at the latest after it has occurred a gynecological examination is absolutely essential, to reconfirm that everything is normal. If it is so, the aches and twinges can be eased or cured with a cup of chamomile tea, drunk very warm, or with peppermint tea or even caraway tea. These three medicinal plant teas contain a great deal of essential oil with a spasmolytic (antispasmodic) effect. Please try them to find which helps you most. You also can employ all three teas in rotation, however.

Preparation of the teas, see page 14.
Application: Drink three cups of tea daily.

Nervous Complaints

● **Tea blends**
The following tea blends have proved reliable for women whose complaints are primarily nervous in origin and who also suffer from insomnia:

Tea Blend 1	oz. (g)
Yarrow, aerial parts	.70 (20)
Lemon balm leaves	.35 (10)
Valerian roots	.35 (10)

Tea Blend 2	
Yarrow, aerial parts	.70 (20)
Lemon balm leaves	.70 (20)
Hop cones	.35 (10)

Tea Blend 3	
Yarrow, aerial parts	.88 (25)
Chamomile flowers	.52 (15)
Valerian roots	.35 (10)
Fennel seeds	.17 (5)

Preparation: Pour 8 ounces (1/4 L) of boiling water over 2 teaspoonfuls of the blend in question, let steep for 10 minutes, then strain.
Application: In a course of treatment lasting several weeks, drink two cups of tea daily. Sweetening with honey is recommended (for diabetics, no sweetening).

Inactivity, Depression

● **Tea blends**

Two tea blends for inactive and depressed women; the blends are quite similar in effect, and you may choose whichever your taste dictates:

Tea Blend 1

Yarrow, aerial parts	.70 (20)
St. John's wort, aerial parts	.70 (20)

Tea Blend 2

Yarrow, aerial parts	.70 (20)
St. John's wort, aerial parts	.35 (10)
Lemon alm leaves	.35 (10)
Orange flowers	.35 (10)

Preparation: Pour 8 ounces (1/4 L) of boiling water over 2 teaspoonfuls of the blend being used, let steep for ten minutes, then strain.

Application: In a course of treatment lasting several weeks, drink two cups of tea daily. Sweetening with honey is recommended (for diabetics, no sweetening).

Leukorrhea

If a medical examination has revealed unmistakably that the leukorrhea, or whitish discharge from the genital organs, is caused neither by a bacterial infection nor by trichomonads or fungi—that is, if it is a constitutional flow—then folk medicine has two time-tested medicinal plants to offer: white dead nettle and lady's mantle, or alchemilla.

For internal application these two medicinal plants can be combined with horsetail, dandelion, and yarrow. For external application, chamomile also has a role to play.

Although we cannot say with certainty which of the substances thus far known to be present in white dead nettle and lady's mantle trigger the effect, their positive effect is repeatedly confirmed by doctors and patients.

External Application

● Tea blends for external application:

Tea Blend 1

White dead nettle flowers	.35 (10)
Chamomile flowers	.35 (10)
Sage leaves	.35 (10)

Tea Blend 2

Chamomile flowers	.35 (10)
Lady's mantle, aerial parts	.35 (10)
Sage leaves	.35 (10)

Tea Blend 3

Chamomile flowers	.35 (10)
Thyme, aerial parts	.35 (10)
White dead nettle leaves	.35 (10)
Erect cinquefoil root	.17 (5)
Lady's mantle, aerial parts	.17 (5)

Preparation: Pour 1 quart (1 L) of boiling water over 2 heaping tablespoonfuls of the blend being used let steep for ten minutes, then strain,

Application: Let the infusion cool, then use it to wash the external genitals. Also suitable for use in sitz baths.

Internal Application

● **Tea blend**

A tea blend for younger women with a weak constitution who suffer from chronic leukorrhea and, at the same time, great nervousness. It is also suitable as an adjunct to medical therapy.

White dead nettle flowers	.35 (10)
Lady's mantle, aerial parts	.35 (10)
Horsetail, aerial parts	.35 (10)
Yarrow, aerial parts	.35 (10)
Lemon balm leaves	.35 (10)
St. John's wort, aerial parts	.35 (10)

Preparation: Pour 8 ounces (1/4 L) of boiling water over 2 heaping teaspoonfuls of the blend, let steep for 15 minutes, then strain.

Application: In a course of treatment lasting four to six weeks, drink one to two cups of tea daily. Sweetening with honey is recommended (for diabetics, no sweetening).

full bath—for a sitz bath, one-third this amount is sufficient. The temperature of the bath water should be between 95 and 98.6°F (35–37°C). Length of bath, 10 minutes. Rest after bathing.

Neurodystonia of the True Pelvis

About 20 percent of the women who visit their gynecologists and complain of various problems—severe, cramplike pain somewhere in the lower abdominal region, often difficult to pinpoint exactly, lower back pain, pain in the breasts before, during, and after menstruation, accompanied by frequent headaches, leukorrhea, and itching that affects the external genitalia—usually are sent home after thorough examination with no serious findings.

In such cases, the versatile yarrow plant has proved helpful in treating the problems.

Yarrow with Dysfunctions

● **Yarrow tea**

I recommend a fairly lengthy (six to eight weeks) course of treatment with yarrow tea.

Preparation: Pour 8 ounces (1/4 L) of boiling water over 2 teaspoonfuls of the aerial parts of yarrow, let steep, covered, for 15 minutes, then strain.

Application: In a course of treatment lasting six to eight weeks, drink one cup of moderately warm yarrow tea daily.

● **Yarrow bath**

To support the tea treatment, I recommend in addition a yarrow sitz bath two or three times a week. In many cases these applications bring marked, sustained improvement.

Preparation and application: Pour 1 quart (1 L) of boiling water over 1.76 to 2.64 ounces (50–75 g) of the aerial parts of yarrow, let steep for 20 minutes, then strain. Add this liquid to a

Menopause

Because menopause (the climacteric), which begins with hormonal changes in a woman, can last for quite a long time, in this chapter recommendations are given for easing the complaints typical of this phase. In contrast to prostate trouble in the male, menopausal complaints disappear on their own after varying lengths of time.

Symptoms and Their Treatment

It frequently happens that women who have led active, well-balanced, optimistic lives suddenly become fearful, irritable, and depressed during menopause, although no pathological organic changes are present. These emotional disorders may be triggered by physical complaints that are due to hormonal change, such as profuse sweating, headaches, and hot flashes. Women with these symptoms feel ill without really being so, for the climacteric is not a disease, but a natural phase of change.

> **Please note**
> When menopause begins, see a gynecologist for a thorough examination, to make sure that all the troublesome symptoms that crop up are completely normal for this stage of life and that no organic disease is present.
> Also ask your doctor about ways to alleviate or to eliminate the symptoms of hormonal change.

I would like to show you some ways to help yourself, ways to use mild herbal remedies to provide more stability, return your disturbed sleep to normal, gradually relieve your anxieties, assuage your irritability and nervousness, and make profuse sweats or headaches more bearable or banish them altogether. A number of medicinal plants lend themselves to these purposes.

Especially effective are St. John's wort, passionflower, valerian, and chamomile. These medicinal plants also are good as accompanying

therapy, if you need to make use of medical help.

> **Please note**
> It is essential to inform your doctor that you intend to treat yourself!

Moodiness

● **Hayseed bath**
Therapeutic baths using lemon balm or lavender may help you, but hayseed baths are especially worth recommending. They provide stability by subduing the overactive autonomic nervous system.
Preparation, see page 25.
Application: One sitz bath or full bath twice a week. Temperature of bath water, 98.6 to 100.4°F (37–38°C), length of bath, ten minutes. Rest after bathing.

● **St. John's wort tea**
Of all the medicinal plants used to treat menopausal complaints, St. John's wort has been the most thoroughly studied. Reports from gynecological hospitals are quite positive. After treatment with tea over a period of four to six weeks, a brightening of the mood is clearly perceptible; nervousness and sleep disturbances diminish; joie de vivre, which had vanished, reappears. For these reasons St. John's wort often is called an herbal "tranquilizer."
Preparation, see page 95.
Application: Drink two to three cups daily.

> **Please note**
> St. John's wort has a photosensitizing effect (sensitivity to sunlight is increased). For this reason, avoid glaring sunlight during the treatment. Ultraviolet light therapy and solarium therapy are not permitted.

● **Tea blends**
Tea blends that contain a high proportion of St. John's wort along with other calming medicinal herbs are no less effective. It is even thought that the medicinal herbs reinforce one another in their effect:

Tea Blend 1

St. John's wort, aerial parts	1.05 (30)
Lemon balm leaves	1.05 (30)
Passionflower, aerial parts	1.05 (30)
Valerian roots	.35 (10)

Tea Blend 2

St. John's wort, aerial parts	.70 (20)
Chamomile flowers	.70 (20)
Lemon balm leaves	.70 (20)
Lavender flowers	.35 (10)
Valerian roots	.35 (10)
Orange flowers	.35 (10)
Rose hips (without seeds)	.35 (10)

Preparation of the tea blends: Pour 8 ounces (1/4 L) of boiling water over 3 teaspoonfuls of the tea blend in question, let steep for five to ten minutes, stirring occasionally, then strain.

Application: In a course of treatment lasting four to six weeks, drink two to three cups of tea daily.

Sleep Disturbances

Difficulties in going to sleep and in staying asleep are among the menopausal complaints that are found especially disturbing and unpleasant. Two tea blends have proved quite beneficial here:

● **Tea blends**

Tea Blend 1
To fall asleep quickly:

Bitter-orange peel	.70 (20)
Valerian roots	.52 (15)
European centaury, aerial parts	.35 (10)
Hop cones	.17 (5)

Preparation: Pour 8 ounces (1/4 L) of boiling water over 2 heaping teaspoonfuls of this blend and let steep for three to five minutes, then strain.

Application: Drink half the tea 30 minutes before bedtime, the rest just before you get in bed.

Tea Blend 2
To prevent early awakening:

Lemon balm leaves	.70 (20)
Valerian roots	.35 (10)
Orange flowers	.35 (10)
Passionflower, aerial parts	.35 (10)

Preparation, see page 14.

Application: Drink one cup of tea just before going to bed. Keep another cup ready in a thermos and drink it slowly when you wake up.

Sweetening the tea with 1 teaspoonful of honey markedly promotes the effect of both tea blends (for diabetics, no sweetening).

Headaches, Profuse Sweating

● **Tea blend**
The following tea is helpful in the treatment of some complaints that appear during the climacteric, such as headaches and profuse sweats.

Speedwell (veronica), aerial parts	.35 (10)
Yarrow flowers	.35 (10)
European cowslip roots	.35 (10)
Sage leaves	.35 (10)
St. John's wort, aerial parts	.35 (10)
Lemon balm leaves	.35 (10)
Valerian roots	.17 (5)
Hop cones	.17 (5)

Preparation and application, see page 14.

Please note
Sage tea, repeatedly recommended for treating the unpleasant spells of profuse sweat, is effective if brewed in a high concentration, but its high tannin content usually makes it hard to digest.

● **Sage tea**

If you would like to try treating sweating spells during menopause with sage tea (please check with your doctor beforehand), then you should use the following method of preparation.

Preparation: Pour 8 ounces (1/4 L) of boiling water over 1 heaping tablespoonful of sage leaves, let steep for ten minutes, then strain.

Application: Drink two cups of tea daily.

● **Mixture of tinctures**

Instead of drinking teas made from medicinal plants, you can also take drops. A mixture of equalizing, calming, and cramp-relieving tinctures of medicinal herbs will help to make the most severe menopausal complaints more bearable or to eliminate them. These tinctures will be mixed for you at some pharmacies or health food stores:

Tincture of St. John's wort (homeopathic original tincture)	.70 (20)
Tincture of passionflower plant (homeopathic original tincture)	.35 (10)
Tincture of oats (homeopathic original tincture)	.35 (10)
Tincture of hawthorn	.35 (10)
Tincture of valerian	.35 (10)
Tincture of chamomile	.35 (10)
Tincture of lemon balm	.35 (10)

Application: As needed, take 10 to 20 drops with sugar (for diabetics, in water) three to five times daily.

● **Mustard powder footbath**

As naturopaths confirm, a footbath prepared with ground mustard also makes a good headache remedy.

Preparation: Put 2 tablespoons of mustard powder, available in pharmacies, into a footbath and pour warm (not hot!) water over it.

Application: Soak your feet in this water for 10 to 15 minutes.

● **Spirit of melissa**

Mention should also be made of the popular spirit of melissa, which is a fine headache remedy.

Application: For internal application, take 30 drops: for external application, dab some on your temples.

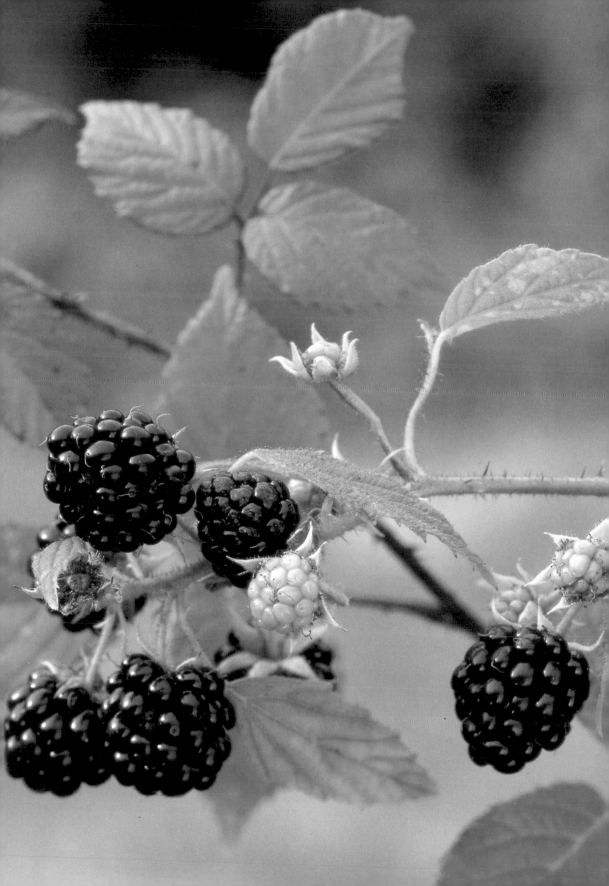

Geriatric Complaints

← *Blackberry*

In Old Age, "A Lot of Things Slow Down"

Vitality, elasticity, spontaneity—qualities we would like to retain as long as we live. It is a fact, however, that with advancing age everything starts to "run a little slower." Our participation in what is going on around us is no longer so lively. We may not be able to adapt to everyday situations as quickly as when we were age thirty. Slight physical infirmities also may make an appearance—our pleasure in eating diminishes, our digestion sometimes is a little off, we catch cold more frequently than usual, and we feel restless and have trouble sleeping.

And naturally we ask ourselves whether we simply have to make the best of these aches and pains or whether there may not be some natural remedies available for them.

Help from Healing Plants

In this chapter you will find medicinal herbal applications that you can use to treat the infirmities and ill health attendant upon old age. I am assuming that you are under a doctor's care, which will ensure that more serious illnesses—which may manifest themselves as slight indispositions at first—are not overlooked.

In the following material you will find suggestions for treatment, which you should please discuss with your doctor. For every medicinal plant application I have given precise instructions; please follow them. As I have said, medicinal plants can be fully effective only if they are appropriately employed, properly prepared, and administered in the exact dose required.

Symptoms and Their Treatment

Lack of Thirst—a Problem in Older People

Older people complain quite often that they have lost all appetite and take no pleasure in eating, but almost no one complains of a lack of thirst. And that gives cause for concern, because many problems such as constipation, diseases of the kidneys and bladder, and even cardiac and circulatory disorders in old age are at least partially attributable to inadequate intake of liquids.

I want to do more than encourage you to drink plenty of liquids, however; I also would like to give you recipes for teas that you can drink as house teas on a regular basis. Tap water and mineral water, as experience indicates, often are not beverages that older people should drink continuously. Wine and beer in large quantities are inadvisable because they contain alcohol and are high in calories; fruit juices generally contain too much sugar and thus too many calories; we know from experience that older people dislike drinking milk in large quantities; and the caffeine content of coffee and black tea is too taxing. A delicious-tasting herbal tea, therefore, is often the remedy of choice.

The ideal daily dose is held to be 2 quarts (2 L) of liquids per day, not counting the soup served with meals or the juice contained in fruits.

How should a tea of this kind be constituted; what requirements does it have to meet?

● **Time-tested tea blends**
A house tea has to taste good and be drinkable either cold or warm. It has to not only look good, but also be easy to digest.

Tea Blend 1	oz. (g)
Raspberry leaves	.70 (20)
Blackberry leaves	.70 (20)
Strawberry leaves	.35 (10)
Rose hips (with seeds)	.35 (10)

Hibiscus flowers	17	(5)
Peppermint leaves	.17	(5)
Pot marigold flowers	.10	(3)
High mallow flowers	.07	(2)

Tea Blend 2

Raspberry leaves	.52	(15)
Blackberry leaves	.52	(15)
Dandelion leaves	.52	(15)
Lemon balm leaves	.35	(10)
Rose hips (with seeds)	.35	(10)
Hibiscus flowers	.35	(10)
Fennel seeds (crushed)	.17	(5)
Red sandalwood	.17	(5)
Pussy-toes (spring cassidony)	.17	(5)
Bitter-orange peel	.17	(5)

Preparation of these tea blends: Pour 1 quart (1 L) of boiling water over 3 slightly heaping tablespoonfuls of the mixture in question, let steep in a covered container for five to ten minutes, then strain. The tea may be stored in a thermos jug.

Application: Several times a day, drink one small cup of tea—2 quarts (2 L) per day are the ideal quantity.

Please note
There are cases in which doctors advise limiting the daily fluid intake. Naturally, the advice of your physician should be followed!

Raspberry, blackberry, and strawberry leaves constitute the basis of the tea in both tea blends, first, because these drugs are largely neutral—that is, they have no specific effect—second, because their taste is reminiscent of black tea. Because continuous use of this basic tea can exacerbate the problems of people who suffer from constipation, rose hips and hibiscus flowers were added. These ingredients produce a tea that generally is easily digestible and also tastes good.

To give the blend eye appeal, several "decorative" drugs are added, including pussy-toes, pot marigold flowers, red sandalwood, and high mallow flowers. Peppermint or lemon balm leaves, fennel seeds, and, not least, bitter-orange peel serve to enhance the taste of these tea blends.

Lack of Appetite: Season Foods Heartily

Loss of appetite usually has its origin in the inactivity and insufficiency of the glands that produce peptic juice in the mouth, stomach, intestines, pancreas, and liver. Disorders in the region of the gallbladder and bile ducts occasionally are the cause. Organic diseases that need treatment are rarely the cause, but the doctor to whom you describe your problems will determine whether any are present. If the loss of appetite is due to old age, then you should first try seasoning your daily diet heartily. The notion that older people need mildly seasoned, bland foods is outmoded—the exact opposite is true. The use of seasonings that taste bitter, aromatic, or spicy is both appropriate and successful for people whose loss of appetite and impaired digestion are caused by old age.

Pepper, mustard, ginger, paprika, curry powder, and nutmeg are permitted, along with those potherbs that taste aromatic and spicy. Not only the digestive organs, but also the heart and circulatory system need the spicy and bitter stimuli in old age. Use of hearty seasonings actually can ease the strain on the heart and circulatory system, which will improve general health. Mustard, pepper, and paprika, once forbidden and viewed as harmful, stimulate the course of almost all the vital processes—in the sense, that is, of increasing vitality. If you want a higher level of vitality, therefore, and thus an enhanced faculty to experience life, you are well advised to season your daily fare heartily, even spicily. In Mexico, where hot chili peppers are highly esteemed and used to flavor a great many dishes, and in the Balkans, where hot paprika is frequently used, heart attacks are far less common than in this country. This is also attributed to the use of spicy seasonings.

A Brief Introduction to Seasonings

If you are well informed about the effect and the use of the individual herbs and spices, I believe you will also be more willing to experiment a bit with seasonings. Be "courageous," then, and prepare your meals—depending on your taste—with spicier, more piquant, and more aromatic seasonings than ever before; eat more healthfully with seasonings.

● Bitter constituents

The bitter constituents of our seasonings first stimulate the taste buds of the retrolingual region. These stimuli are transmitted to the receptive end organs (receptors), and the secretion of gastric juices is initiated. As a result, the entire digestive system is excited to activity. Because in seasoning the emphasis is on enhancement of taste, however, we choose not the classic herbal bitters, such as gentian or European centaury, but those that introduce sufficient bitter qualities yet still possess a pleasantly aromatic taste. Summer savory, basil, marjoram, thyme, wormwood, and mugwort are the recommended seasonings if you are interested in improving the performance of your digestive tract.

● Spicy constituents

The spicy substances in our seasonings are no less beneficial to health than the bitter constituents. They promote the flow of saliva to a special degree, stimulate gastric motility (movement), and ensure that the foods ingested do not lie "like a rock in the stomach" for an excessive length of time. They stimulate peristaltic motion and improve the mixing of the enzymes and partially digested food in the intestines. Further, spicy seasonings—as I mentioned previously—have a favorable influence on the function of the circulatory organs. They lessen the strain on the circulatory system as it performs its role in the task of digestion. No serious experiment has been able to prove that spicy seasonings cause damage to the kidneys, for example, as is so often alleged. Overdoses are ruled out in any event, because an excess of spicy seasonings spoils the dish. One little side effect of liberal use of paprika has become apparent: Older men who have trouble urinating because of benign prostate enlargement can tell some improvement.

Among the spicy seasonings, from which you can choose as your taste dictates, my own favorites are pepper, paprika in various degrees of hotness, moderately hot chili peppers, turmeric, allspice, galingal, nutmeg, ginger, radish, and mustard in various degrees of hotness.

● Essential oils

The essential oils in our herbs and spices serve primarily to improve taste, which is, after all, the purpose of using seasonings. Cinnamon, vanilla, rosemary, lemon balm, peppermint, clove, star anise, and citrus fruits probably serve this purpose exclusively (these seasonings are available in herb and spice shops, and health food stores).

There are, however, other seasonings containing essential oil that have a specific effect; they can cure flatulence, a feeling of fullness, and cramplike abdominal pain. These "healing" herbs and spices include dill, anise, fennel, caraway, and coriander. They all are botanically classified as Umbelliferae (Apiaceae) and contain large amounts of essential oils that vary in composition but have quite similar effects. These effects are described as digestive (improving digestion), spasmolytic (helping to relieve cramps), and carminative (causing the release of stomach or intestinal gas). If you know that certain foods generally cause you to have gas pains, then these are precisely the seasonings you should use frequently. Caraway and coriander are the most effective. Among the foods that many people do not digest easily—a problem that can become increasingly pronounced in old age—are dishes containing sauerkraut and cabbage, vegetable stews, and fresh bread. Usually whatever amount of seasoning suits your taste will be sufficient to relieve flatulence.

Digestive Complaints

Unwellness After Eating

● **Caraway tea**

If generous use of seasonings does not eliminate a feeling of unwellness after eating, caraway tea is sure to help you.

Preparation: Pour 8 ounces (1/4 L) of boiling water over 1 heaping teaspoonful of caraway seeds that have been freshly crushed in a mortar or coarsely ground in a spice mill, let steep, covered, for about five minutes, then strain. Please do not sweeten!

Application: Drink one cup of tea immediately before or directly after eating.

● **Coriander tea**

Coriander also can be helpful; if you prefer it to caraway, you should drink coriander tea.

Preparation and application, as for caraway tea.

● **Tea blend**

If you are one of those people who dislike both caraway and coriander as single teas, I recommend a tea with the following makeup:

Chamomile flowers	1.05 (30)
Caraway seeds (crushed)	.70 (20)
Lemon balm leaves	.70 (20)
Coriander seeds (crushed)	.35 (10)
Peppermint leaves	.35 (10)

Preparation: Pour 8 ounces (1/4 L) of boiling water over 1 heaping teaspoonful of this blend, let steep, covered, for about five minutes, then strain. Please do not sweeten!

Please note

A special type of flatulence—accumulations of gas in the epigastric region that force the diaphragm upward and constrict the heart—resembles attacks of angina pectoris: paroxysmal, constricting pain in the cardiac region. Caraway tea or coriander tea can help here, too. To determine the actual state of affairs, however, you must consult a physician.

The following tea blends have proved reliable, particularly for older people; try them all to see which is best for you.

Feeling of Fullness

● **Tea blend**

Especially helpful after meals:

Peppermint leaves	.35 (10)
European centaury, aerial parts	.35 (10)
Caraway seeds (crushed)	.35 (10)
Caraway flowers	.35 (10)

Inability to Digest Fat

● **Tea blend**

Especially well suited for people who have trouble digesting fat:

Thyme, aerial parts	.70 (20)
Peppermint leaves	.35 (10)
Mugwort, aerial parts	.35 (10)
Yarrow, aerial parts	.35 (10)
Bitter-orange peel	.35 (10)

Lack of Appetite

● **Tea blend**

European centaury, aerial parts	.35 (10)
Chamomile flowers	.35 (10)
Lemon balm leaves	.35 (10)
Rose hips (with seeds)	.35 (10)
Angelica root	.17 (5)
Gentian roots	.17 (5)
Ginger rhizome	.17 (5)

Preparation of these tea blends: Pour 8 ounces (1/4 L) of boiling water over 2 teaspoonfuls of the blend being used, let steep for five minutes, then strain.

Application: As needed, drink 1 cup of tea before meals—in sips and as warm as possible. Please do not sweeten.

Gastric Trouble

● **Tea blend**

Many older people suffer from gastric problems that are found after medical examination not to be based on any underlying diseases. With these complaints, which vary greatly in form and intensity and thus cannot be described precisely, this tea has proved reliable:

Lemon balm leaves	.88 (25)
Chamomile flowers	.88 (25)
European centaury, aerial parts	.35 (10)
Bitter-orange peel	.35 (10)
Orange flowers	.35 (10)
Hop cones	.35 (10)
Valerian roots	.35 (10)
St. John's wort, aerial parts	.35 (10)

Preparation: Pour 8 ounces (1/4 L) of boiling water over 2 heaping teaspoonfuls of this blend, let steep three to five minutes, stirring repeatedly, then strain.

Application: At the outset drink one cup of tea three times a day; depending on the complaint, gradually switch over to one or two cups of tea daily; finally, drink one cup of tea only as needed.

Constipation

Chronic constipation, from which more women than men seem to suffer, is a common affliction in older people. By no means should you immediately resort to the use of laxatives or popular medicinal plants such as senna, rhubarb, alder buckthorn, and aloe. Continuous use of laxatives results in depletion of the body's electrolytes with all its corollary forms of damage, including cardiac and circulatory problems, muscle cramps, and disordered cell metabolism. Constant use of laxatives may results in colitis. The user also may become dependent on laxatives for initiating elimination. It is preferable to stimulate the intestinal tract in another way.

● **Little pointers**

You may be helped by a few little, but important, pointers that I have often passed on to my customers at the pharmacy, who also have found them helpful as a rule.

In your daily diet, give preference to foods that are high in roughage, including high-fiber vegetables, sauerkraut, cabbage dishes, potatoes, salads made from wild greens, and coarse-textured fruits; eat coarse-grained whole-wheat bread instead of white bread; drink plenty of liquids (see page 112), preferably herbal teas or juices that you press yourself, unsweetened if possible; ensure that you get sufficient exercise regularly; and, above all, "listen" to your intestines. At the first indication that your bowels are ready to move, go to the toilet. If you neglect to do so, the body will withdraw additional moisture from the stool, which will become hard and more difficult to eliminate.

● **Flaxseed**

An effective herbal remedy with which you can help "train your bowels to be regular" is flaxseed; it swells up in the intestinal tract and triggers an expansion stimulus that sets off peristalsis, which in turn results in evacuation.

Application: Three times a day, take 1 to 2 heaping teaspoonfuls of rough-ground flaxseed (linseed or flaxseed meal) with at least 1 pint (1/2 L) of water—without prior soaking.

● **Tea blend**

A healthful house tea for people who suffer from constipation:

Hibiscus flowers	1.05 (30)
Rose hips (with seeds)	1.05 (30)
Raspberry leaves	.35 (10)
Blackberry leaves	.35 (10)
Lemon balm leaves	.17 (5)
Peppermint leaves	.17 (5)

Preparation, see page 14.

Application: Drink up to 1 quart (1 L) of tea per day.

● **Tamarind pulp**

One very well-tried home remedy is tamarind pulp, pharmaceutically known as *Pulpa Tamarindorum*. This is the pulp of the ripe fruits of the tamarind tree (*Tamarindus indica*). The high content of fruit acids is responsible for the mild laxative action—the pulp contains malic acid, succinic acid, citric acid, and tartaric acid. The effect is bolstered by the plentiful amounts of invert sugar and the potassium bicarbonate present in the pulp.

Application: In the evening, take 1 tablespoon ful of tamarind pulp; alternatively, take 2 teaspoonfuls twice a day.

● **Prunes**

In conclusion, I would also like to recommend prunes. Soften 10 to 20 prunes in water in the morning, then eat them, together with the liquid in which they have soaked, before going to bed.

Diarrhea

Older people complain about diarrhea far less often than about constipation. Self-help with medicinal plants, however, is possible only in cases where diarrhea appears after eating too large a meal or unsuitable foods.

Important: With diarrhea of all types, copious amounts of body fluids are lost, along with salts, electrolytes, and sugar. For this reason, visit your doctor without delay.

● **Tea blend**

I recommend a tea blend that you can use to bring quick, long-lasting relief in severe cases. If no effect is apparent after two days at most, you need to consult a physician:

Erect cinquefoil roots	1.41 (40)
Thyme, aerial parts	1.05 (30)
Chamomile flowers	.70 (20)
Peppermint leaves	.35 (10)

Preparation, see page 14.

Application: Drink three to five cups of tea daily. Please do not sweeten.

Sleep Disturbances—Restlessness—Mild Depressions

Older people very frequently suffer from these complaints. They may feel quite well otherwise and have no organic diseases, but—as they tell us repeatedly—they are afraid of the night because they are unable to sleep. Sometimes it takes them a long time to fall asleep, sometimes they wake up after a brief sleep; always they experience the state of lying awake and the gloomy thoughts and worries that torment them then are extremely wearing.

Sleep Disturbances

● **Examine your daily routine**

In such cases, please don't reach for some strong medicine, because it is definitely not healthy to forcefully bring about sleep through anesthetization and achieve tranquility through stupefaction. I don't even recommend that you try an herbal tea remedy at first, but rather that you take a close look at your daily routine. Possibly the "little snooze" that has become a habit in the afternoon is getting so long that you are simply not yet tired by evening. An evening stroll may help you, or bedtime reading may help to induce sleep. It may also be that you are one of those people who get by on less and less sleep, often on fewer than six hours. As for the "gloomy thoughts" and worries, please make a conscious effort not to take them with you to bed and into the night. The advice of an old gentleman may help you. He recommends that immediately after the evening meal you call to mind a pleasant event from bygone days and "keep it in remembrance" before going to bed, in order to "play" with it there, recalling details or reexperiencing the event as more pleasurable than it was in actuality. This is a pleasant activity, but it will tire you at the same time. There are many possible ways to find your way back to sleeping well. You may think of others that work better for you.

● **Sleeping drink**

If everything you try is of no avail, however, and sleep still is slow in coming, then a sleep-inducing drink might be the right remedy.

I recommend that you do as many older people in the Romance language-speaking countries do; they drink chamomile tea with milk.

Preparation, see page 21; mix the prepared tea with milk (one part of milk to three parts of tea).

Application: Shortly before going to bed, drink one cup of tea with milk, sweetened with 1 teaspoonful of honey. (Diabetics may take the sleeping drink only if it is unsweetened.)

● **Tea blends**

The following teas also have a good effect. Try them to see which helps you most and tastes best.

Tea Blend 1

Lemon balm leaves	.35 (10)
Valerian roots	.35 (10)
Chamomile flowers	.35 (10)
Orange flowers	.35 (10)
Rose hips (with seeds)	.35 (10)
Lavender flowers	.35 (10)
Hop cones	.35 (10)

Tea Blend 2

St. John's wort, aerial parts	1.05 (30)
Hawthorn flowers	.70 (20)
Lemon balm leaves	.70 (20)
Chamomile flowers	.35 (10)
Hop cones	.17 (5)

Preparation of the tea blends, see page 14.

Application: Before going to bed, drink one cup of tea; if you wake up at night, drink one additional cup of tea, sweetened with honey (for diabetics, without honey).

Please note

Waking up during the night is often a reaction to too little blood sugar. For this reason, it may be useful to eat a small sugar lozenge or a little piece of milk chocolate when you awake. This applies also to diabetics, who absolutely must consult their physician in advance, however. If the doctor approves, he or she will also specify how much may be eaten.

● **Soothing baths**

Soothing baths are often-used, effective aids to sleep. These have proved reliable: lemon balm baths, hop baths, lavender baths, valerian baths, and hayseed baths.

Preparation and length of the baths, see page 25.

● **Herbal pillow**

An herbal pillow may also be a highly effective aid to falling asleep and staying asleep, particularly for older people. Of the many possible mixtures of medicinal plants that may be used to fill your herbal pillow, I would like to recommend the following:

Hop cones	1.05 (30)
St. John's wort, aerial parts	.70 (20)
Lavender flowers	.70 (20)

Preparation and application: Sew a small bag of fine linen with edges measuring approximately 4 x 4 inches (10 x 10 cm) to 6 x 6 inches (15 x 15 cm). Provide one side with a zipper. Loosely fill the bag with enough of the herb mixture to make a plump pillow (don't fill it to bursting). The filling usually will remain effective for one month.

Place the herbal pillow either under your customary pillow or under the bed covers. You can also lay your head directly on it, however (in this case, put it in a pillowcase). It is also possible to place the pillow on your chest; this way you will inhale the "healing aromas" during the night.

Mild Depressions

Many older people often feel lonely and abandoned; they feel unwell or ill-tempered, brood a great deal, and are virtually unable to be really glad about anything, even if they have all the reason in the world. They themselves describe their state as mildly depressed and often feel unable to find a way out of this sadness and sense of loneliness.

● **Tea blend**
Such time-tested medicinal plants as lemon balm and St. John's wort are useful precisely in mild depressions of this kind. A tea made from these two medicinal herbs will bring improvement after some time, in the sense of brightening your mood.

Preparation, see page 14.

Application: In a course of treatment lasting at least six weeks, drink two to three cups of tea daily.

With mild depressions, as described above, an herbal pillow also can do you good; just try it sometime.

Decline in Cardiac Activity

If you notice that climbing stairs is not as easy as it used to be, and if you get "out of breath" on walks when you go uphill, then you should not immediately despair. These are declines in the performance of your heart that may occur in old age. In many people these problems are fairly severe, in others, barely perceptible.

Please note
By all means, please see a doctor for a thorough heart examination before you treat yourself with a medicinal plant application!

Sometimes the doctor will initiate treatment with heart-strengthening preparations made from species of foxglove (*Digitalis*), often with mild-acting medicinal plant therapies as well, because there are excellent teas that strengthen the heart "weakened by age" when used in a course of treatment. The results are improved supply of oxygen and glucose (sugar) to the heart muscle and improved circulation in the coronary vessels.

Myocardial Insufficiency

● **Hawthorn tea**
First place in the ranks of effective medicinal plants goes to hawthorn. Its flowers or a blend of its flowers and leaves (in a 1:1 ratio) yield a heart-strengthening tea suitable for long-term use. Hawthorn has been thoroughly studied by scientists, and it is acknowledged to be effective in treating incipient myocardial insufficiency, particularly in the area of the coronary vessels and the heart muscle; feelings of pressure and constriction in the heart area; insufficient pulse rate; and cardiac arrhythmia.

Preparation, see page 14.

Application: In a course of treatment lasting several weeks, drink one cup of tea two to three times daily.

People who are treated with hawthorn tea feel fresher, can climb stairs more easily again, and notice on their walks that they can handle slight inclines without shortness of breath and without tiring quickly. These patients also report that they sleep better and wake up less frequently during the night.

Nervousness

● **Tea blend**
Another medicinal plant that has been known for many years as a remedy for heart disease is motherwort (*Leonurus cardiaca*). Its effect is similar to that of valerian, that is, calming and relaxing.

For this reason I recommend mixing motherwort with lemon balm and hawthorn if you are concerned primarily with calming a "nervous heart." The bitter-orange peel in the following tea blend serves as a tonic, that is, it strengthens and stimulates. The blend has proved highly reliable:

Hawthorn flowers	.70 (20)
Motherwort, aerial parts	.70 (20)
Lemon balm leaves	.70 (20)
Bitter-orange peel	.35 (10)

Preparation: Pour 8 ounces (1/4 L) of boiling water over 1 to 2 heaping teaspoonfuls of this blend, let steep for 20 minutes, then strain.

Application: In a course of treatment lasting several weeks, drink one cup of tea two to five times daily. You may sweeten the cup of tea in the evening with honey. (Diabetics drink their tea unsweetened in the evening also.)

High Blood Pressure

Elevated blood pressure, particularly in older people, is usually considered "normal." I would like to contradict this widespread opinion!

> **Please note**
>
> In every case, elevated blood pressure has to be treated by a doctor! Please have your blood pressure checked regularly.

Slightly elevated blood pressure (systolic blood pressure from 140 to 159 mm Hg and diastolic pressure from 90 to 94 mm Hg) can be treated with hawthorn tea—only with your physician's consent—at least on a trial basis.

● **Tea blend**

I recommend that you give the following tea a try—under a doctor's supervision!

Hawthorn leaves and flowers	1.05 (30)
Valerian roots	.17 (5)

Preparation, see page 14.

Application: Drink two cups of tea daily.

Overly Low Blood Pressure

Overly low blood pressure readings, relatively rare in older people, are uncommonly trouble-some because efficiency is substantially lessened as a result.

> **Please note**
>
> In every case, overly low blood pressure has to be treated by a doctor. Please have your blood pressure checked regularly.

● **Rosemary tea**

Rosemary tea also finds application in folk medicine, as a remedy for low blood pressure.

Preparation: Pour 8 ounces (1 (4 L) of boiling water over 1/2 teaspoonful of rosemary leaves, let steep for ten minutes, then strain.

Application: Drink two cups of tea daily.

● **Rosemary bath**

Rosemary baths are also helpful in stimulating the heart and circulatory system. *Preparation and length of bath*, see page 123.

Strengthening the Heart and Circulatory System

● **Tea blend**

A time-tested tea for strengthening the heart and circulatory system, particularly in older people:

Hawthorn leaves and flowers	.75 (21.5)
Raspberry leaves	.75 (21.5)
Rosemary leaves	.65 (18.5)
Rose hips (with seeds)	.65 (18.5)
Motherwort, aerial parts	.51 (14.5)
Bitter-orange peel	.24 (7)
Pot marigold flowers	.08 (2.5)

Preparation: Pour 8 ounces (1/4 L) of boiling water over 2 teaspoonfuls of this blend, let steep for about five minutes, then strain.

Application: Drink two to three cups per day.

Chronic Cough (Old Age Cough)

As a result of asthma, chronic bronchitis, and pulmonary emphysema (abnormal distention of the lungs), a chronic cough in old age is so common that the name "old age cough" is applied to it in Germany. With smokers, we speak of "smoker's cough" in this connection. Whatever it is, all efforts to ease it must be preceded by a medical examination, because successful therapy is impossible without a diagnosis.

Please note
Always let your doctor determine the causes of a cough and specify the treatment.

Asthma does not respond well even to intensive treatment, because chemical agents are also unable to effect a cure. In such cases your doctor will have no objection to the use of herbal teas as an adjunct to medical therapy, as they are extraordinarily effective.

Secretional Obstruction of the Bronchial Tubes

There are many medicinal plants that have proved helpful with older people in treating coughs and congestion and disinfecting the bronchial tubes. I recommend several well-tried tea blends.

Tea Blend 1

Iceland moss	1.05 (30)
High mallow flowers	.35 (10)
Mullein flowers	.35 (10)
Thyme, aerial parts	.35 (10)

Tea Blend 2
A tea that is even better at loosening the viscid mucus:

Iceland moss	1.05 (30)
European cowslip roots	.70 (20)
Lemon balm leaves	.35 (10)
Thyme, aerial parts	.35 (10)
English plantain, aerial parts	.35 (10)

Preparation of the tea blends: Pour 8 ounces (1/4 L) of boiling water over 2 heaping teaspoonfuls of this blend, let steep in a covered container, stirring occasionally, for five to ten minutes, then strain.
Application of the tea blends: Before going to bed in the evening drink one large cup of tea,

sweetened with 1 tablespoonful of honey (diabetics have to drink the tea unsweetened). Place the tea in a thermos jug on the bedside table. In the morning drink one cup of tea about half an hour before getting up.

● **Tea blend**
In conclusion I would like to mention a tea for colds that is effective precisely with the cough so common in old age.

Linden flowers	.35 (10)
Elderberry flowers	.35 (10)
Lemon balm leaves	.35 (10)
Chamomile flowers	.35 (10)
Thyme, aerial parts	.35 (10)

Preparation, see page 14.
Application: In a course of treatment lasting several weeks, drink two to three cups of tea daily.

Prostate Trouble

In old age—though in some men it begins as early as age forty-five—the prostate gland enlarges. Because the prostate encircles the urethra at the place where it emerges from the bladder, any enlargement or swelling interferes with urination. At first the increase in size is scarcely noticed, but later the stream of urine becomes weaker and the bladder is no longer emptied completely. With prostatic enlargement, the growth of the prostate frequently ceases in a stage at which the discomfort can be eased with mild medicinal plants to such an extent that it is barely perceptible. The enlarged gland, however, will not decrease in size. There are also malignant enlargements of the prostate (cancer), which today can be treated successfully if detected early enough.

Please note
Please have regular checkups to see whether cancer of the prostate is present. The earlier a cancer is detected, the greater are the chances of a cure. If you notice any problems in urination, if your bladder is not

emptying completely, then please go to the doctor, who will take the necessary measures.

Difficulty in Urinating

● **Stinging nettle tea**

You can use medicinal plant teas as a suitable adjunct to the doctor's measures. I recommend stinging nettle, dandelion, quaking aspen (*Populus tremuloides*) buds, and—with reservations—also small-flowered willow herb. Although stinging nettle may be used as a single tea (made from the leaves; even more effective if made from the roots), dandelion and quaking aspen buds are found primarily in tea blends.

Preparation of stinging nettle tea from leaves, see page 72.

Preparation of stinging nettle tea from roots: Pour 8 ounces (1/4 L) of cold water over 2 heaping teaspoonfuls of stinging nettle roots, bring slowly to a boil, let boil for about one minute, let steep for about 10 minutes, then strain.

Application of both kinds of tea: Drink three to four (up to five) cups of tea per day.

● **Tea blends**

Two additional tea blends are in my opinion also suitable for application in mild cases of benign prostatic enlargement (also called benign prostatic hyperplasia, BPH).

Tea Blend 1

Stinging nettle roots	1.05 (30)
Quaking aspen buds	.35 (10)
Dandelion roots	.35 (10)

Preparation: Pour 8 ounces (1/4 L) of cold water over 2 heaping teaspoonfuls of this blend, bring to a boil, let steep for five minutes, then strain.

Application: In a course of treatment lasting two to three weeks, drink two to three cups of tea daily.

Tea Blend 2

Dandelion roots (with aerial parts)	.70 (20)
Stinging nettle leaves	.70 (20)
Chamomile flowers	.70 (20)
Lemon balm leaves	.70 (20)
Peppermint leaves	.35 (10)

Preparation, see page 14.

Application: Drink three cups of tea daily. This tea may also be drunk as a house tea at the onset of prostate trouble.

● **Small-flowered willow herb**

I mentioned that I can recommend small-flowered willow herb for treating benign prostatic hyperplasia only with reservations. This medicinal plant was greatly overrated in folk medicine, and so little is known about it that I cannot in good conscience advise you to apply this medicinal herb. If your doctor has a different opinion, you can prepare a tea from small-flowered willow herb as described on page 14. The application is the same as for stinging nettle tea.

● **Pumpkin seed treatment**

A pumpkin seed treatment for benign prostatic hyperplasia, however, is highly recommended. The effect has been confirmed, although the reason for it cannot yet be explained fully. The voiding of urine is eased, the stream of urine grows stronger, and urination is no longer interrupted. Less residual urine remains in the bladder, and the feeling of pressure in the bladder and urethra is no longer experienced as unpleasant. No findings on retrogression of the prostatic enlargement are available.

Application: Several times a day, take 1 tablespoonful of hulled pumpkin seeds.

Unfortunately, the seeds of our garden pumpkins and squashes have little effect. The pumpkin seeds used for medicinal purposes, specially bred for application with prostate trouble, are available in health food stores.

"Gout" in Old Age

Perhaps you are familiar with these conditions—you want to get up from your chair, but it's not so easy to do because the small of your back hurts; you want to walk, but it takes a few steps for you to get into your stride; you want to make a vigorous reach for something and feel a stabbing pain in your joints. All this may, but need not, be rheumatism; for this reason people often talk about "gout." This term is used to include all these transitory aches and pains in the muscles and joints, usually the result of signs of degeneration associated with old age. In serious cases, of course, medical treatment is unavoidable, but by and large you can manage with medicinal plant treatment in the form of tea therapy or medicinal herbal baths.

Please note
Before beginning treatment with medicinal plants, a medical examination is necessary to determine the causes of the complaints.

Again and again people ask whether and how they can use medicinal herbal teas to get relief and whether it is suitable to supplement medical therapy with teas. The last question should be put to your doctor—although I believe I can predict his or her answer: an unequivocal yes.

We can ease rheumatism, but not cure it. Neither chemical nor herbal remedies have that power. For this reason, everything that gives relief is accepted by physicians, provided it does no harm.

Before I recommend teas for you, I would like to deal with the juniper berry treatment, which in my experience is extremely popular, precisely with older people. This treatment is not devoid of problems, because with a high dose of juniper berries the possibility of considerable irritation of the kidneys is not to be ruled out. However much the treatment is praised, I cannot recommend it in this case!

Pain in the Joints

● **Dandelion tea**
My favorite among the medicinal plants that help to ease pain in the joints, or arthralgia, is dandelion. I advise eating plenty of dandelion greens in springtime salads and using it at least three times a year in a course of treatment with dandelion tea.

Preparation: Pour 8 ounces (1/4 L) of cold water over 2 heaping teaspoonfuls of dandelion roots with the aerial parts, bring slowly to a boil, keep at the boiling point for about one minute, let steep for about ten minutes, then strain.

Application: In a course of treatment lasting six to eight weeks, drink two to three cups of tea daily.

● **Tea blend**
If you want to upgrade the taste of the tea, which admittedly is not particularly good, try the following blend:

Dandelion roots (with aerial parts)	1.05 (30)
Rose hips (with seeds)	.35 (10)
Hibiscus flowers	.35 (10)
Peppermint leaves	.35 (10)

Preparation, see page 14.
Application: In a course of treatment lasting six to eight weeks, drink two to three cups of tea daily.

● **African devil's claw**
Also successful in long-term treatment to alleviate rheumatic complaints is African devil's claw (*Harpagophytum procumbens*), native to southern and southwestern Africa. Its rhizome, prepared as a tea, is often employed to treat articular rheumatism. Usually you can buy the drug already packaged in health food stores and some pharmacies. The enclosed directions for use should be followed to the letter.

More and more people are ascribing a very positive effect to devil's claw in the treatment of digestive disturbances—especially in older people—and calling devil's claw tea a remedy for premature aging. Please do not expect too much of this tea—miracle drugs simply don't exist.

Herbal Baths to Invigorate and Relax

The latest research has taken "the wind out of the sails" of all those who asserted that baths were effective—if at all—only by virtue of their pleasant warmth, and that all additives were mere gimmicks. Scientists at the University of Munich's Institute of Medical Balneology and Climatology succeeded in proving that essential oils in bath water are resorbed by the skin and that even minerals—albeit to a more modest degree—enter the body in this way. In addition, during the bath active substances can be taken in through inhalation, and definite healing stimuli can be triggered by the olfactory nerve.

Also significant in this connection is the research performed by Professor Müller-Limroth on the efficacy of hayseed applications. He was able to prove that baths and poultices improve circulation in tissue, strengthen connective tissue, and allay pain.

Herbal baths, therefore, are not only a pleasure, but also a source of healing. Generally you buy herbal baths (medicinal bath additives; please pay close attention to the directions) in pharmacies and health food stores, which is simpler and more convenient than preparing bath additives yourself. If you would like to do just that, however, you will learn how in the following section.

Please note
Medicinal baths may strain the heart and circulatory system and, with venous problems, are not always appropriate. For this reason, please get your doctor's advice before applying medicinal baths.

Soothing

● **Valerian bath**
Pour 2 quarts (2 L) of water over 3.52 ounces (100 g) of valerian roots (valerian tea), bring to a boil, let boil down for about ten minutes, then strain. Add the extract to the bath water. You can also add 3.52 ounces (100 g) of tincture of valerian to a full bath.

Temperature of bath water, 95 to 100.4°F (35–38°C), length of bath, 10 to 15 minutes. Rest after bathing.

● **Lemon balm bath**
Pour 5 quarts (5 L) of boiling water over 2.11 to 2.46 ounces (60–70 g) of lemon balm leaves, let steep for about 20 minutes, then strain. Add the extract to the bath water.

Temperature of bath water, 95 to 100.4°F (35–38°C), length of bath, 10 to 15 minutes. Rest after bathing.

● **Hop bath**
Pour 2 quarts (2 L) of water over 1.76 ounces (50 g) of hop cones, bring to a boil, let steep for about 20 minutes, then strain. Add the extract to the bath water.

Temperature of bath water, 95 to 100.4°F (35–38°C), length of bath, 10 to 15 minutes. Rest after bathing.

● **Lavender bath**
Pour 1 quart (1 L) of water over 1.76 to 2.11 ounces (50–60 g) of lavender flowers, bring to a boil, let steep for 20 minutes, then strain. Add the extract to the bath water.

Temperature of bath water, 95 to 100.4°F (35–38°C), length of bath, 10 to 15 minutes. Rest after bathing.

● **Rosemary bath**
Pour 1 quart (1 L) of water over 1.76 to 2.11 ounces (50–60 g) of rosemary leaves, bring to a boil, let steep for ten minutes, then strain. Add the extract to the bath water.

Temperature of bath water, 95 to 100.4°F (35–38°C), length of bath, 10 to 15 minutes. Rest after bathing.

Easing Pain, Improving Circulation

● **Hayseed bath**
Pour 5 quarts (5 L) of water over 10.58 to 17.63 ounces (300–500 g) of hayseed, bring to a boil, let boil down for about five minutes, then strain. Add the extract to the bath water.

Temperature of bath water, 95 to 100.4°F (35–38°C), length of bath, 10 to 15 minutes. Rest after bathing.

● **Horsetail bath**

Soak 1.76 ounces (100 g) of horsetail (aerial parts) in 2 quarts (2 L) of hot water for about one hour, briefly bring the mixture to a boil, then strain. Add the extract to the bath water.

Temperature of bath water, 98.6 to 100.4°F (37–38°C), length of bath, 10 to 15 minutes. Rest after bathing.

● **Yarrow bath**

Pour 2 quarts (2 L) of water over 7.05 ounces (200 g) of yarrow (aerial parts), bring to a boil, let boil down for ten minutes, then strain. Add the extract to the bath water.

What you need to know

The hayseed bath and the yarrow bath are also suitable for easing tension during menopause (see page 107). The rosemary bath is also felt to be helpful with rheumatism.

Handy Pointers

● For dry skin, rubbing in oil of St. John's wort is helpful.

● With a dry mouth, anise is helpful. You can chew the ground seeds, but you also can suck strong anise candies.

● Warts often will disappear if you rub castor oil into them several times a day.

● With ulcerated legs (*Ulcus cruris*), healing is stimulated by compresses made with arnica tea or calendula flower tea.

Preparation of the teas: Pour 8 ounces (1/4 L) of boiling water over 1 heaping teaspoonful of the drug in question, let steep for 10 minutes, then strain.

Application of the teas: Soak multilayered gauze in the lukewarm tea, lay it on the places to be treated, and secure with a gauze bandage. The compress has to be replaced several times a day.

● An ointment dressing with arnica or calendula is also to be recommended. If reddening of the skin, accompanied by itching and/or burning, results, you are one of those people who are allergic to arnica or (more rarely) calendula. Treatment should be discontinued at once.

● The development of bedsores (decubitus ulcers) in bedridden patients can be prevented by rubbing the problem areas (heels, base of the spine, back) with calendula ointment several times a day.

● Fruit vinegar taken with sugar can help to get rid of hiccups. (Diabetics should not try this application.) According to a doctor from Boston, however, a sure cure is eating a slice of lemon on which you have dripped 20 drops of Angostura bitters.

● Chronic headaches will vanish if you take a warm footbath two or three times a week, with 2 tablespoonfuls of mustard powder added to the water. Length of bath, 10 to not more than 15 minutes.

● A "stale taste" in your mouth, usually in conjunction with bad breath, can be remedied with tea made from fenugreek seeds.

Preparation: Pour 8 ounces (1/4 L) of cold water over 1 teaspoonful of ground seeds, let the mixture stand for six hours, then bring it briefly to a boil and strain.

Application: Gargle and rinse your mouth.

● Pressure sores caused by dentures heal quickly if you rub them several times a day with tincture of myrrh. Often it suffices just to rinse your mouth daily with lukewarm water to which tincture of myrrh has been added: 30 drops to one glass of water.

● Stinging nettle seeds steeped in fortified wine are a tonic for older people of either sex. You can make the tonic yourself.

Preparation: Pour 1 quart (1 L) of fortified wine over 1.76 ounces (50 g) of stinging nettle seeds, set aside for 10 days, then strain.

Application: In a course of treatment lasting eight weeks, take 1 to 3 tablespoonfuls of tonic daily.

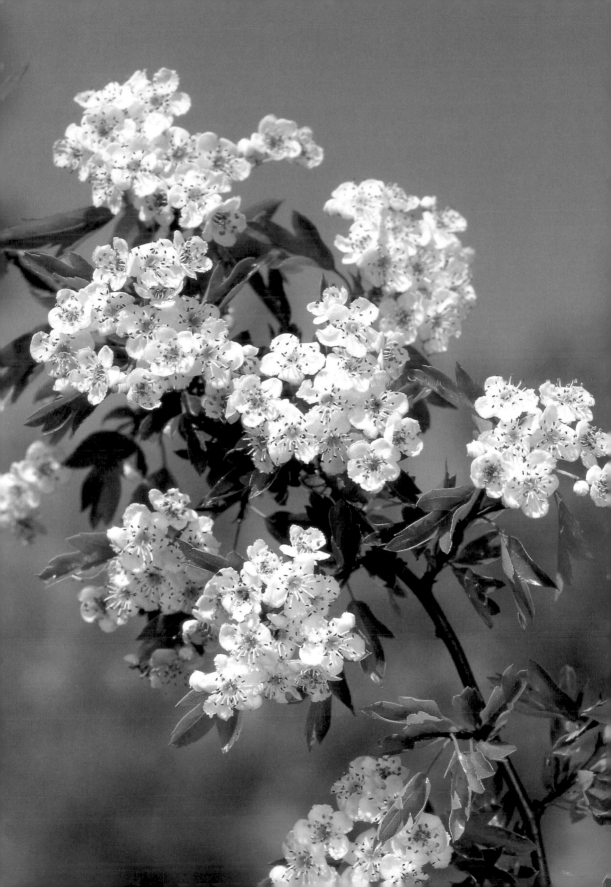

Cardiac and Circulatory Disorders

← *Hawthorn*

Healing Plants in the Treatment of Heart Trouble

Without exception, patients with demonstrably diseased hearts belong in a doctor's care. Herbal tea applications, however, can be quite useful in treating damage to the heart and circulatory system caused by excessive strain, damage that results from the hectic pace of modern life, excessive demands in school or at work, and, very often, unhealthful habits as well. These are the cases in which medical examinations have produced no evidence of cardiac pathology, yet the functional capacity of the heart is impaired. Nervous agitation, occasional palpitations, decreased tonicity, rapid tiring, and—as it is often described—"running out of breath" while exerting oneself by climbing stairs or performing physical labor are the complaints. The cause is insufficient circulation of blood to the heart muscle, which results in a diminution of functional capacity. Often it is also a vascular change, arteriosclerosis (hardening of the arteries). In these cases, you can achieve improvement of these complaints through medicinal teas, but their primary effect is preventive. The hearts of older people are by nature no longer functioning at full capacity and require some support, so that the infirmities of old age (decline in performance, nervous agitation, palpitations, angina pectoris, difficulty in breathing, hypertension, and edema, or dropsy) can be postponed or made less noticeable. The efficacious herbal tea treatments are outstandingly well suited for this purpose.

After recovering from illnesses, especially infectious illnesses, but also after operations, the convalescent phase is extremely lengthy in many people. They can't quite seem to get back on their feet, and they feel lethargic and tired, although they have gotten over their illness. Here something is amiss with the circulatory system, and blood pressure is often too low. In these cases, medicinal plants—after consultation with your doctor—offer their services for therapy.

Not least, let me also mention that many physicians offer patients recovering from heart attacks (myocardial infarctions)—along with numerous suggestions regarding their future lifestyle and prescriptions for the necessary medications—advice about also using hawthorn flower tea to prevent a second attack, suggesting that this tea be drunk as a good follow-up therapy. Hawthorn flowers are extremely well suited for exercising a beneficial effect on the heart, however damaged it may be. Muscular efficiency is increased, the coronary vessels are expanded, and circulation is improved, with the result that the oxygen supply of the heart and the entire organism is markedly better. In addition, hawthorn flowers, as Professor Dr. R. F. Weiss also points out clearly, have no side effects, even when used in a tea over a long period of time.

I would like to place motherwort, valerian, and lemon balm alongside hawthorn in a supporting role. Hops, too, with its calming effect, and St. John's wort must be mentioned in this connection. Rosemary and lavender will stand you in good stead as tonic herbal baths for the treatment of circulatory problems, in particular, low blood pressure.

What You Need to Know

Today, diseases of the heart are treated to a large extent with active substances derived from medicinal plants, primarily from plants that we classify as poisonous.

Most important here is digitalis therapy, treatment with glycosidic active substances from the various species of foxglove (*Digitalis* species).

Admittedly, it is not medicinal teas made from these plants that we use, but fine-tuned, standardized finished preparations and isolated pure substances in the form of drops, tablets, capsules, suppositories, or injections.

In some cases the active ingredient, after being isolated and purified, has been subjected to analysis and, finally, has been successfully synthesized.

Symptoms and Their Treatment

For Prevention

● **Hawthorn flower tea**

Among the medicinal plants listed, hawthorn is the one I recommend also as a single drug (that is, unblended) for treatment of cardiac and circulatory complaints. Anyone who while still young is under continuous pressure to achieve or feels overtaxed by physical or intellectual labor has to expect that this excessive demand will have a negative effect on his or her heart. Even if you are conscious of nothing yet, if you think your heart is still sound as a bell because you have noticed neither palpitations (tachycardia) nor heart constriction (stenocardia) in yourself, even if your blood pressure is normal and the EKG readings are satisfactory, it is not too soon for you to start drinking hawthorn tea as a preventive measure, without any misgivings. Hawthorn eases the strain on the overworked heart and improves the supply of oxygen to the heart muscle, thus preventing signs of degeneration. With good reason, hawthorn is considered an excellent preventive of the dreaded myocardial infarction. And, as stated, aging and old people can use hawthorn to keep their hearts healthy to a large extent, allay existing problems, and halt the progress of arteriosclerosis (hardening of the arteries).

Preparation: Pour 1 cup of hot water over 1 heaping teaspoonful of hawthorn flowers, let steep for 15 minutes, then strain.

Application: In the morning or after breakfast, drink one cup of tea in sips, and drink a like amount before going to bed. The evening cup of tea also helps you to go to sleep and promotes nighttime regeneration. It is especially good to sweeten the tea in the evening with 1 teaspoonful of honey (for diabetics, no sweetening).

Nervous Agitation, Feelings of Oppression

● **Tea blend**

If you suffer from nervous agitation and feel constricted and oppressed (angina pectoris), if you feel that you're not getting enough air, or if you break into a sweat at slight exertions, you should try the following tea:

	oz. (g)
Hawthorn flowers	1.05 (30)
Motherwort, aerial parts	.35 (10)
Lemon balm leaves	.35 (10)
Valerian roots	.17 (5)

Preparation: Pour 1 cup of boiling water over 1 heaping teaspoonful of the tea blend, let steep for ten minutes, then strain.

Application: Drink one cup of tea, lukewarm and in sips, in the morning and evening.

Flatulence

● **Tea blend**

People whose heart and circulatory system are weakened frequently complain of flatulence, although they have no gastric disease or digestive disorders. These gas pains (meteorism), which are found quite unpleasant, are eased by the following tea:

Hawthorn flowers	1.05 (30)
Lemon balm leaves	.35 (10)
Chamomile flowers	.35 (10)
Caraway seeds	.35 (10)

Preparation: Pour 1 cup of boiling water over 1 heaping teaspoonful of the blend, let steep for ten minutes, then strain.

Application: Drink one cup of tea, lukewarm and in sips, in the morning and evening.

Dejection

For patients with cardiac insufficiency who are not only nervous, but also dejected, morose, lacking in volition, or even depressed, a tea made with St. John's wort is appropriate:

Hawthorn flowers	1.05 (30)
St. John's wort, aerial parts	1.05 (30)
Lemon balm leaves	.70 (20)

Preparation: Pour 1 cup of boiling water over 1 heaping teaspoonful of the blend, let steep for ten minutes, then strain.

Application: Drink one cup of tea, lukewarm and in sips, in the morning and evening.

Circulatory Insufficiency

● **Tea blend**

All people who want to stimulate their circulatory systems, including "tired" adolescents, all convalescents—especially if recovering from infectious diseases—and older people with slightly low blood pressure, will do well to prepare a tea containing lemon balm and rosemary. Here I usually recommend a few additional ingredients:

Rosemary leaves	.70 (20)
Lemon balm leaves	.70 (20)
Rose hips (with seeds)	.35 (10)
Hibiscus flowers	.35 (10)

Preparation: Pour 1 cup of boiling water over 1 heaping teaspoonful of the blend, let steep for ten minutes, then strain.

Application: Drink one cup of tea, lukewarm and in sips, in the morning and evening (not during pregnancy!).

Herbal Baths for Relaxing and Easing Tension

I can recommend three medicinal plants that have proved highly reliable: valerian, lemon balm, and rosemary.

● **Valerian bath**

It calms the nervous heart and has a sedative effect. If you take a valerian bath before going to bed, you will fall asleep quickly and easily. The effect of this bath is so compelling that you may fall asleep in the bathtub (for this reason, be cautious!).

Preparation: Pour 3 quarts (3 L) of water over 3.52 ounces (100 g) of valerian root, boil for about ten minutes, then strain. Add the liquid to the bath water.

Instead of this you also can add 7.05 ounces (200 g) of tincture of valerian to the bath water. Ready-made valerian bath extracts are available in some pharmacies and health food stores.

Application: Temperature of bath water, 98.6°F (37°C), length of bath, 10 to 15 minutes. Rest after bathing.

● **Lemon balm bath**

This bath has an equalizing effect, and with nervousness it acts as an antispasmodic.

Preparation: Pour 1 quart (1 L) of water over 1.76 to 2.11 ounces (50–60 g) of lemon balm leaves, bring to a boil, and strain after ten minutes.

Ready-made lemon balm bath extracts are also available in pharmacies and health food stores.

Application: Temperature of bath water, 98.6°F (37°C), length of bath, 10 to 15 minutes. Rest after bathing.

● **Rosemary bath**

This bath is prized especially by hypotonics (people with overly low blood pressure) and by patients with peripheral circulatory disturbances. **DO NOT USE DURING PREGNANCY!**

Preparation: Pour 1 quart (1 L) of water over 1.76 to 2.11 ounces (50–60 g) of rosemary leaves, bring to a boil, and strain after ten minutes.

Application: Temperature of bath water, 98.6°F (37°C), length of bath, 10 to 15 minutes. Rest after bathing.

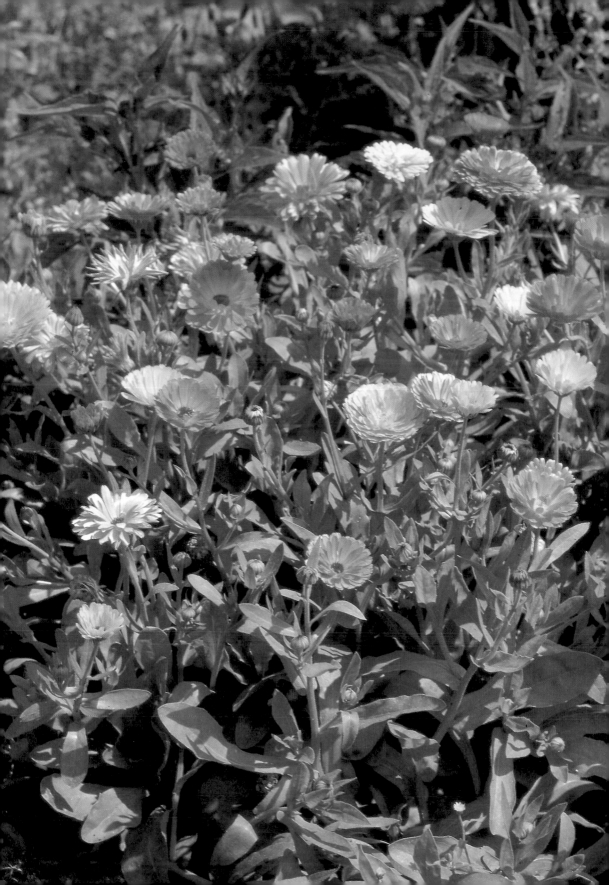

Minor Injuries, Skin Irritations

The Proper Healing Plants for Use with Injuries and Wounds

← *Calendula*

The Proper Healing Plants for Use with Injuries and Wounds

Injuries happen quickly in sports. More serious injuries, such as torn tendons or broken bones, make a trip to the doctor essential on account of the severe pain alone. Usually, however, the injuries are harmless ones that you can treat yourself.

With the right medicinal plants, these less serious injuries are quickly healed.

In addition, there are wounds that heal poorly, and they also respond well to treatment with medicinal plants.

If you are now convinced that the number of plants I am going to offer will be enormously large, I have to disappoint you. My favorites, the ones with which I can get along, are arnica, comfrey, chamomile, and pot marigold.

Symptoms and Their Treatment

Swellings

● **Damp arnica compresses**

These compresses bring quick relief with all swellings that are caused by sports mishaps or appear following sprains, dislocations, strains, and contusions. These swellings usually are accompanied by considerable pain.

An arnica compress can also assuage the pain of swellings that arise after bone fractures, which of course require treatment by a physician. A room-temperature to cool arnica compress stimulates circulation, so that effusions of blood are resorbed more quickly and varicose ulcers heal better.

There are two ways to make the solutions for arnica compresses. First, arnica tea may be used for the compress; second, a dilute tincture of arnica may also be used for a damp compress.

Preparation of the arnica tea for the compress: Pour 8 ounces (1/4 L) of boiling water over 1 heaping teaspoonful of arnica flowers, let steep, covered, for five minutes, then cool to room temperature.

Application: Soak multilayered bandaging gauze (or cotton) with the warm tea, place the gauze around or on the area to be treated (the swelling or the wound), and wrap a gauze bandage around it. It is important that the bandage remain permeable to air (do not cover with plastic wrap). If the liquid has evaporated, you can dampen the bandage again by pouring more liquid on it. Changing the dressing is not necessary.

Tincture of arnica for compresses: You can get this in pharmacies under the name of *arnica tinctura* (tincture of arnica).

Application: Add 1 teaspoonful of tincture of arnica to 8 ounces (1/4 L) of water at room temperature (in a bowl). Apply the damp compress as described above for the arnica (tea) compress.

> **Warning**: Arnica is a violent poison when taken internally—keep all arnica products, including the dried flowers, out of the reach of children and pets. Any unused tea for compresses should be flushed down the sink, immediately.

Please note

Some people have an allergic reaction to arnica compresses. The areas that have been treated turn red and begin to itch, and in the worst case, blisters may form. With reactions of this kind, discontinue treatment at once.

Arnica ointment, available in pharmacies and health food stores, is effective in the treatment of venous problems, rheumatism, sciatica, and blunt sports injuries (not open wounds). No objection can be raised to this application (unless an allergy is present!). Please read the package enclosure carefully, however.

Minor Sports Injuries

● **Comfrey compresses**

The medicinal plant known as comfrey is used to treat relatively minor sports injuries. With this plant, however, the root is boiled for a while and the resulting decoction is used for compresses.

Preparation of the solution for comfrey compresses: Pour 8 ounces (1/4 L) of cold water over 2 teaspoonfuls of comfrey root, bring to a boil, let steep for five minutes, then strain.

Application: As for arnica compress, see page 134.

For wounds that are healing poorly, comfrey ointment (pharmacy and health food store) is appropriate, along with the damp compress. The active substance allantoin liquefies pus and necrotic tissue and thus promotes healing.

Bedsores

● **Pot marigold compresses**

Pot marigold (or calendula) is the third medicinal plant that I like to recommend in the form of a compress or an ointment for the treatment of sports injuries, particularly to people who are allergic (skin irritations) to arnica preparations. Pot marigold usually is tolerated better, although allergic reactions are not entirely out of the question here, too.

Preparation of the calendula infusion for the compress: Pour 8 ounces (1/4 L) of boiling water over 1 heaping teaspoonful of pot marigold flowers, let steep, covered, for five minutes, then strain and let cool to room temperature.

Application: As for arnica compress, page 134.

Pot marigold has proved particularly reliable in the treatment of bedsores (decubital ulcers) in seriously ill, bedridden patients (intensive care) or in old age. For this purpose, cover the affected areas on the skin once a day with a layer of calendula ointment (pharmacy) the thickness of the back of a knife blade. Application over time leads to improvement or healing of existing open sores.

To prevent bedsores, treatment with calendula ointment is recommended. In addition to turning the patient frequently, spread calendula ointment on the endangered areas.

Application: Treat the areas in question with calendula ointment at least three times daily.

Cramped Muscles

● **Chamomile compress**

Chamomile is known everywhere as a vulnerary (wound-healing) herb. Less well known is the fact that a chamomile compress can relax cramps in muscles (also in the back) and thus can be helpful in the treatment of sports injuries. It is easy to make and to apply.

Preparation of the chamomile extract for the compress: Pour 1 quart (1 L) of boiling water over 5 tablespoonfuls of chamomile flowers, let steep for 15 minutes. After being strained, the chamomile extract is ready for use.

Application: Thoroughly dampen a small towel with the hot chamomile extract, squeeze it out, and place it, as warm as possible, on the area to be treated. Wherever possible (for example, on the hands, feet, arms, and legs) secure the towel with a gauze bandage. Periodically—about ten times in 30 minutes—dampen the compress with some hot chamomile extract. Then conclude the treatment and apply oil of St. John's wort to the reddened skin (available in pharmacy and health food stores).

Handy Pointers

● Insect bites: If you have been stung by mosquitoes, horseflies, bees, or wasps, for example, the area around the sting site should be rubbed immediately with crushed yarrow leaves. This will reduce the itching and the swelling.

● With inflammations of the gums and the mucous membranes of the mouth and throat, and with pressure sores caused by wearing dentures, the medicinal plant sage is helpful. Sage tea (*Preparation*, see page 109) used as a gargle several times a day has a healing and anti-inflammatory effect.

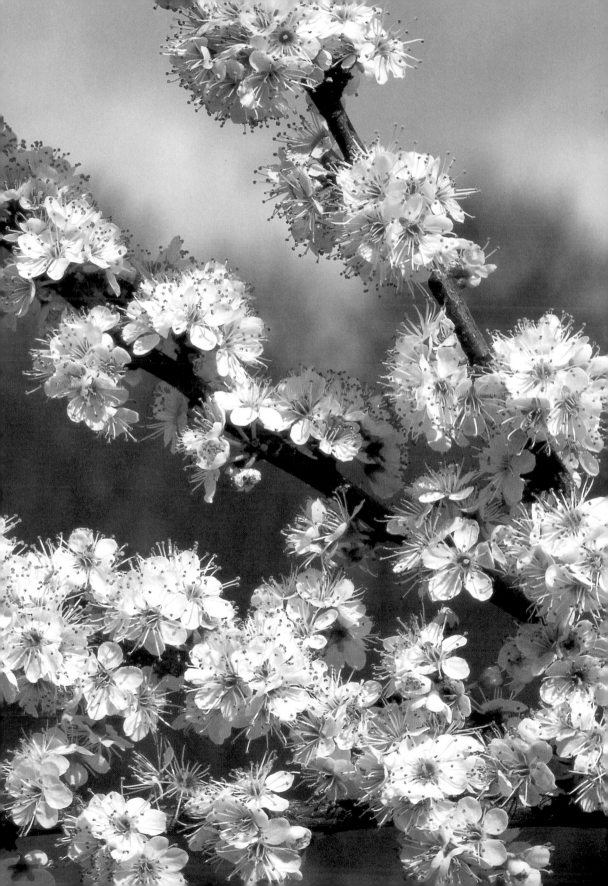

Compendium of Medicinal Plants

← *Sloe or Blackthorn*

Becoming Familiar with Healing Plants

I would like you to become more closely acquainted with the healing plants recommended in this book. Then you will understand that my tea recommendations take into account all that is presently known about the effect of the medicinal plants used in the teas—knowledge based on scientific research or long years of experience. I have also included historical information of interest. All the medicinal plants recommended in this guide are introduced to you in alphabetical order by their common name, so that you can find your way about as quickly as possible.

Cultivating Medicinal Plants

Please also note the last section of each medicinal plant profile; there I have indicated whether you can raise the medicinal plant in question yourself, and if so, how it should be grown and tended in your garden or in tubs on your balcony or patio.

You will acquire detailed knowledge of any medicinal herbs you raise yourself, and at the same time you can also enjoy the flowers, the fragrance, or the plant as a whole.

Proper Harvesting and Careful Preparation

I have compiled some important rules for harvesting your medicinal herbs; they are applicable unless other instructions are given in the text.

For harvesting and drying medicinal plants, the following rules apply:
● Harvest only the part of the plant that is used for pharmaceutical purposes (given in the profile).
● Never harvest in rain, fog, or damp weather; the material you collect will spoil. The best time for harvesting is morning, after the dew has dried.
● Harvest only clean plants. Dust and dirt lessen the quality, because medicinal plants should not be washed.
● Harvest leaves when they are young, but completely developed; flowers, when they have just bloomed or shortly before they bloom; entire plants (all aerial parts), at the beginning of the blooming season; fruits and seeds, when they are completely ripe.
● The drying of the material you collect should be viewed as preservation. In this process the plant's own enzymes are deactivated, and bacteria, viruses, and fungi are deprived of their nutritive medium. Drying should be done carefully and quickly. You can dry the plants in the open air, on screens that allow air flow from above and below; you can tie them into bunches and hang them up to dry (in a warm, well-ventilated place); or you can dry them in artificial heat (kitchen oven with its door open). With aromatic herbs—plants rich in essential oil, the flowers or leaves of which are used (for example, lemon balm or peppermint)—the drying temperature should not exceed slightly more than 95°F (35°C). All other plant parts, such as the bark, coarse leaves and stems, and fruits and seeds, can tolerate temperatures up to about 122°F (50°C).
● It is advisable to cut up the dried plant parts and briefly dry them once more. Then put them in containers that can be tightly closed, protected from light and dampness, for proper storage (see page 12).

Medicinal Plants From A to Z

African Devil's Claw: Native to South Africa

In the 1960s, a healing drug that made headlines came from South Africa. It was extolled as a miracle drug that promised to cure rheumatism, diabetes, and diseases of the stomach, gallbladder and liver. Ten to 15 years later nothing more was heard of this medicinal plant, because it failed to meet people's expectations—that is, it did not perform miracles. Today we know that these hopes had some basis in fact. Thanks to its anti-inflammatory properties, African devil's claw serves as a soothing agent in the treatment of rheumatic diseases; with indispositions in the sphere of the digestive organs it is used as bitters.

African devil's claw (*Harpagophytum procumbens*) is classified as one of the Pedaliaceae, which are related to our foxglove species.

The original plant has a large knobby root, from which fresh shoots break forth every year at the beginning of the rainy season. The shoots hug the ground and reach a length of 39 to 78 inches (1–2 m). The stalked, opposite leaves grow about 2 to 3 inches (5–7 cm) long and about 1 to 1.6 inches (3-4 cm) wide; they are fleshy, oval, and often deeply sinuous at the margins. Fruits that quickly lignify develop from large, trumpet-shaped violet flowers. The fruits have long, branched arms that are equipped with barbed hooks. These burr fruits are crushed and distributed by the stamping of feet; they become caught in the hooves of grazing animals and are spread in this way.

The healing drug, however, is obtained not from these unusual capsules, but from the storage tubers of the roots, which are dug up after the blooming season. Dried and cut into fairly small pieces, these tubers are sold under the name of harpagophytum tea or African devil's-claw tea. Scientists are making great efforts to study the effect of African devil's-claw tea, to

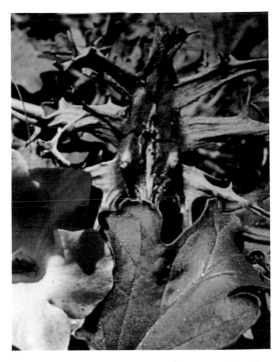

African Devil's claw

get a clear understanding of the operational mechanism of its components. The soothing effect of African devil's-claw tea when used to treat arthrosis (diseases of the joints) and its calming effect on the digestive process in the stomach and intestines, however, can be viewed as confirmed.

Devil's claw should not be used during pregnancy.

Cultivation
Raising this plant yourself is not possible in our latitudes.

Angelica: Stimulates the Flow of Gastric Juice

Angelica is considered an "outsider" among the medicinal herbs that are used to treat stomach and intestinal problems, but anyone who is familiar with the plant knows its value in treating lack of appetite, dyspepsia, flatulence, and

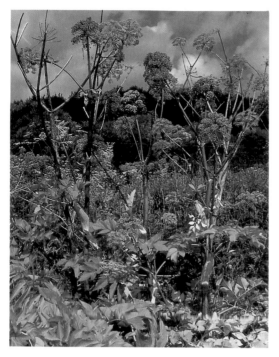

Angelica

Botanists, who call this medicinal plant *Angelica archangelica*, place it in the carrot family (Apiaceae-Umbelliferae). Angelica is native to northern Europe. It is more common in Scandinavia, Greenland, and Iceland than on the coasts of the North Sea and the Baltic, where it is relatively scarce. It grows in cool, damp meadows, but also in the valleys of low mountain ranges. It certainly was unknown to the Greeks and Romans. *Angelica atropurpurea* (Purplestem angelica), a North American native, has similar properties and uses.

Angelica, a stately plant, is able to reach a height of about 6-1/2 feet (2 m). The grooved, hollow stem is occasionally purplish at the top of the plant. The leaves have enlarged convex sheaths at the base of the leafstalks and have two to three pinnate parts. They become smaller toward the top of the plant and are less clefted. The upper part of this herb is branchy. At the branch ends grow the inflorescences, 20- to 40-radiate double umbels with bristly small involucral leaves. The tiny greenish-white flowers smell of honey.

The medicinally useful parts—the angelica roots—come almost exclusively from cultivation.

Please note

Angelica belongs to the Apiaceae = Umbelliferae, a family with many poisonous members that can be mistaken for this medicinal plant. Do not collect angelica yourself under any circumstances!

Cultivation

Angelica can be grown in your garden or on your balcony. A northern plant, it will do best in the cooler regions of the United States and in Canada. Seeds are available through catalogs, but you will be more successful if you can obtain young plants at a nursery. Grow in well-drained, slightly acid soil. Angelica will do best in a moist, partially shaded location. After the second year, you can propagate with offshoots and root cuttings. Roots can also be harvested in early fall of the second year.

the sensation of fullness. Preserved in honey, angelica is also esteemed as a tonic, particularly for older people. Chewing the root is recommended even for people suffering from a hangover after excessive alcohol consumption.

Pharmacists call this medicinal plant *Amara aromatica*, a bitter, aromatic drug, and view it, like all other medicinal plants that contain essential oil and bitter constituents, as a proven stomachic that also acts on the intestinal tract. For this reason, the German Office of Health recommends the use of angelica root for problems such as a feeling of fullness, flatulence, and mild, cramplike gastrointestinal pain, caused by underproduction of gastric juice, for example.

Please note

If you plan to use angelica for a fairly long time, you will have to dispense with ultraviolet or tanning salon treatments as well as exposure to strong sunlight for the duration. This drug will render you sensitive to light.

Arnica: Threatened with Extinction

In its native habitat—that is, in unfertilized or only slightly fertilized alpine pastures and heathland at medium elevations, occasionally in flat country as well—arnica is commonly known also as mountain tobacco and leopard's bane. There it ranks first among the healing herbs. Its flowers generally are used to prepare an extract known as spirits of arnica, a solution in alcohol of an essential principle, for treating (see page 136) sprains, bruises, rheumatism, strains, and wounds that are slow to heal. This medicinal plant has also been used internally in folk medicine, in the form of "arnica drops," for example, to benefit people suffering from lack of appetite and gastric, intestinal, cardiac, and menstrual pain, but this treatment is dangerous and not recommended.

Please note

I want to issue a clear warning against internal use. Consumption of arnica preparations can cause serious damage to the heart as well as painful irritation of the stomach and intestines.

Today arnica is used only externally. The German Office of Health recommends arnica-based preparations in the form of ointments, tinctures, and infusions to treat strains, bruises, sprains, crush injuries, and muscle and joint pain, as well as arnica compresses to promote the healing of wounds. Arnica ointment is recognized as beneficial in the treatment of tired legs, swellings, and rheumatic pain.

Botanists call arnica *Arnica montana* and assign it to the botanical family of the composites (Asteraceae = Compositae). It is an attractive plant that charms every hiker and nature lover in early summer when it displays its bright yellow flowers.

The close heads of florets with their surrounding wreath of bracts are never completely regular, which makes the flower so extraordinary. Arnica is a perennial; it has a rhizome that creeps horizontally in the soil. The coarse, hairy stem reaches a height of up to about 20 inches

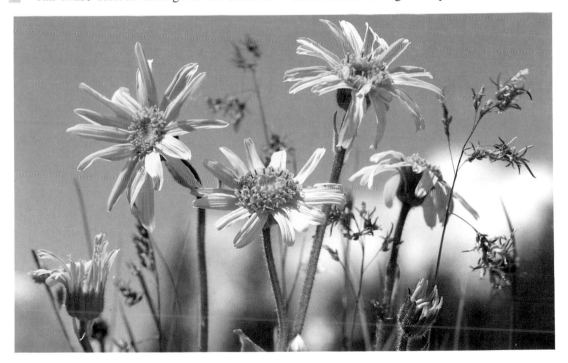

Arnica

(50 cm). It grows from a basal rosette that hugs the ground, and it bears one to two pairs of smaller stem leaves and a terminal flower (inflorescence), below which two additional rudimentary flowers grow in the axils of the upper pair of leaves. The yellow flower heads, or capitula, are surrounded by a two-rowed involucre of bracts covered with short, shaggy hairs. The labiate flowers have three tiny teeth. Recently *Arnica chamissonis*, meadow arnica, was approved as a drug supplier in addition to *Arnica montana*, which cannot be cultivated profitably and whose wild populations are almost completely exhausted. Its effect is quite similar to that of *Arnica montana* and it is easier to raise.

Please note
Arnica is threatened with extinction. For this reason, it is on the list of strictly protected plants. Please respect this. Even if your grandmother and great-grandmother made their own spirits of arnica from plants they collected themselves, you should refrain from doing likewise—for the sake of Mother Nature.

Cultivation
Any attempt to grow arnica in your garden is not likely to succeed. I advise against it unless you are a hobby gardener with a great deal of experience. In the larger seed stores you can buy packets of seed with instructions for cultivating seedlings.

Basil: The "Royal's Herb," Well-known and Loved

Is it a healing herb or a seasoning? This question is often asked, but the answer is that aromatic, spicy potherbs such as basil are both.

I recommend basil, also known as sweet basil, primarily as a seasoning that older people in particular can use to stimulate their stomach and their entire digestive tract. Foods seasoned with basil are digested faster and better, the flow of gastric juices in the stomach is given a stimulus, and the appetite is improved. With approval of the German Office of Health, basil in the form of a medicinal tea is used as a supportive therapy to relieve flatulence and the sensation of fullness.

The origin of this herb is uncertain. It may have come from South Asia, but today it is cultivated as a perennial in various subspecies, strains, and varieties in the subtropics and tropics. From the Mediterranean basil, crossed the Alps to our herb garden (it can be cultivated easily, even in balcony and window boxes). Among the numerous common names, the terms gentleman's herb and royal herb indicate the popularity of this plant, and the name German pepper emphasizes that basil is a spicy, aromatic herb.

The leaves may be used fresh or dried to flavor soups, stews, cheese, fish, ground meat, fried potatoes, or poultry that is high in fat (geese, ducks).

Ocimum basilicum, as botanists call it, is an annual herb belonging to the mint family (Labiatae = Lamiaceae). This bushy plant has

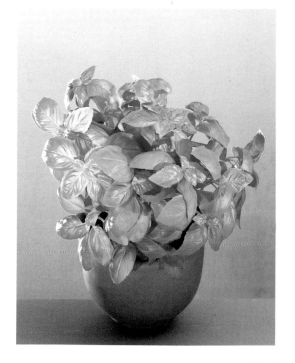

Basil

numerous branches and grows about 20 inches (50 cm) tall. The stalked, ovate leaves are entire-margined or slightly toothed. White, pink, red, or scarlet flowers grow in axillary cymes (false umbels).

Cultivation

Where winter temperatures fall below freezing, seeds should be sown outdoors only after mid-May. Sow the seeds at intervals of 8 to 12 inches (20–30 cm). Basil prefers sandy, loamy soil. Because it needs light to germinate, the seeds should merely be pressed down lightly, not covered with earth. The seed will sprout after 10 to 14 days. The only care required consists of weeding, hoeing, and plentiful watering in case of dryness.

Basil also can be grown easily in balcony boxes or flowerpots filled with sandy, loamy soil. To this potting soil add some mineral fertilizer (one thimbleful per pot). In a sunny spot sheltered from wind, the plants will flourish well, and you will have fresh basil on hand at all times. Ensure yourself of a supply for the winter by cutting the plants off about 2 to 4 inches (5–10 cm) above ground level shortly before they bloom, tying them into bunches, and hanging them up to dry. Store them in metal boxes, protected from light and dampness.

Bean Hulls: Popular in Folk Medicine

More correctly known as bean pods, they are the dried hulls of our common, garden or kidney, bean, with the seeds removed. The bean, known to botanists as *Phaseolus vulgaris*, belongs to the bean family (Fabaceae = Leguminosae).

In folk medicine two primary areas of application are given for bean pods; they are used to prevent the formation of gravel and urinary calculus and to treat diabetes. I have to reject the tea as a remedy for diabetes, however, because no measurable successes have turned up. Nevertheless, the chromium, arginine, and silicic acid content appears interesting for science as well. Whatever research during the next few years may bring to light, today I consider it irresponsible to propose treating diabetics with bean hull

tea. However, the tea is an appropriate means of preventing renal gravel and renal calculus (kidney stones). This is also acknowledged by the German Office of Health, inasmuch as the following appears on the circular enclosed in the package, under the heading "Areas of Application": Increases quantity of urine; for prevention of the formation of urinary gravel and urinary calculus.

Cultivation

Beans are raised in vegetable gardens. The seed is available in seed stores; the packet includes directions for cultivation. Beans need nourishing garden soil and a sunny location.

Bearberry: A Disinfectant for the Bladder and Kidneys

In contrast to other popular medicinal plants, bearberry has no long history of therapeutic use: Doctors became aware of it only in the mid-

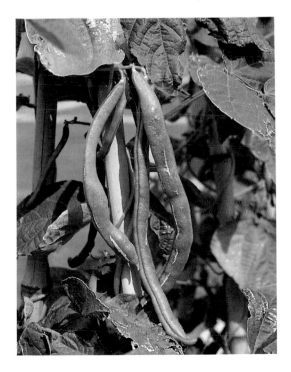

Bean Hulls

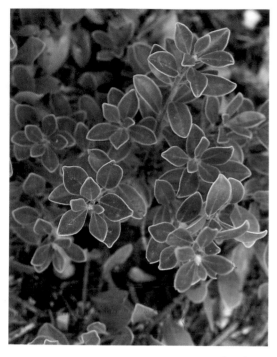

Bearberry

plant foods; however, because bearberry leaves usually are employed in acute cases, one would like to make the urine alkaline as quickly as possible. This can be done by adding 1/2 teaspoonful of baking soda (bicarbonate of soda) to the tea. One additional factor needs to be considered—the extremely high tannin content of bearberry leaves. If the tannin is present at full strength in the tea, it will heavily tax the digestive tract. This can be remedied easily by preparing the tea with cold water. Bearberry leaves also contain flavonoids, hydroquinones, and iridoids.

Arctostaphylos uva-ursi is the botanical name of bearberry, which belongs to the heath family, or Ericaceae. It is a low-growing evergreen shrub that produces long branches, which in turn put forth roots once more. Thus one finds extensive mats of considerable density. The leathery leaves are thick and coarse, usually obovate but occasionally spatulate as well. On their upper sides a network of veins is clearly visible. In contrast to the leaves of the lingonberry (*Vaccinium vitis-idaea*), the undersides of bearberry leaves are not covered with tiny brown dots. The small bell-shaped or jug-shaped flowers of the bearberry shrub are white, with rose-pink tips. When ripe, the racemes, which have few flowers in each cluster, develop round red berries that, unlike lingonberries, are inedible, though they are not poisonous.

The leaves, the only parts used for medicinal purposes, can be harvested year-round, but they are most efficacious in late summer. The bearberry leaves available commercially come exclusively from wild populations as a naturalized introduced plant.

eighteenth century. In the early nineteenth century it was considered to be a medication, and today it is mentioned in many pharmacopoeias.

Bearberry leaves, also popularly known as *uva-ursi*, are a time-tested medicine for treating infections in the area of the kidneys, the bladder, and the urinary passages. If used promptly, a tea made from bearberry leaves can relieve acute problems in no more than three days. The German Office of Health recommends bearberry-leaf tea for supportive treatment of bladder and kidney infections, but warns against prolonged application because continued use can result in hydroquinone poisoning. It also is not necessary to drink it for longer periods, because acute bladder and kidney catarrhs generally will disappear within a few days after treatment with bearberry-leaf tea.

The primary active substance is listed as arbutin. That is correct, of course, but first the actual effective component, hydroquinone, has to be released from it. This requires urine that shows a slightly alkaline reaction. Over time that can be achieved by means of a diet rich in

Cultivation

Purchase several plants at a garden center and set them in humus-rich garden soil. The plants will strike root quickly and later will put forth trailing shoots that take root. You can start additional plants from them in pots. Set five to six (up to eight) plants per 1.19 square yards (1 m).

After only two or three years, the plants you have set will cover as much as 70 to 80 percent of the planted area; later, growth will slow down considerably. Only the leaves are harvested, which is possible year-round, but you should not begin harvesting them until the first bloom.

Birch: Its Leaves Stimulate Urine Production

In Slavic and Germanic tradition the birch tree has played a special role. It was believed that by being whipped with a birch rod before sunrise on Easter Sunday a person could "barter for" health, and that diseases could be transferred to birch branches; witches were said to ride birch brooms at their gathering on the Brocken in the Walpurgis night. Even in the absence of superstition, however, birch has retained its magic. At Pentecost and on Corpus Christi Day, house entrances are decorated with birch branches; birches are planted along country roads; and the birch is also common in yards and gardens.

In addition to the leaves, other parts also had medicinal uses: the bark and the "birch water," the sap of young birch trees, which was tapped in spring and made into an alcohol-based hair lotion. What remains of these applications is primarily the use of a tea made from birch leaves as a remedy for bladder and kidney ailments, as a depurative (blood purifier), and as a source of relief from rheumatic complaints in the broadest sense. Birch leaves are a beneficial component of numerous teas used as to purify the blood and to treat bladder and kidney problems and rheumatic and metabolic disorders.

The German Office of Health recommends birch leaves to stimulate urine production, to treat diseases where increased urine production is desirable (for example, gravel), and to prevent urinary calculus.

> **Please note**
> Birch leaves may not be used to treat edema (collections of fluid) resulting from reduced cardiac and renal activity.

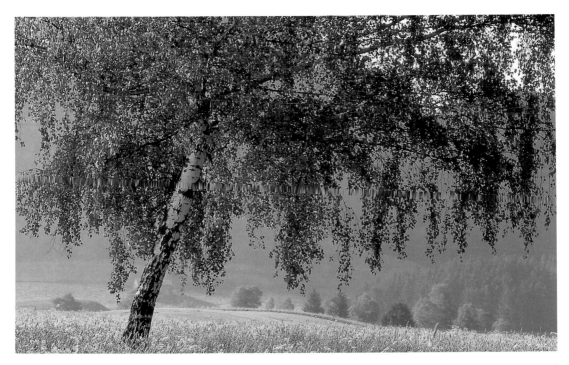

Birch

We use the leaves of both the marsh birch (*Betula pubescens*) and the silver birch (*Betula pendula*). The leaves are collected and dried in spring (see page 138).

Cultivation

If you bring a small sapling home from the nursery, within only a few years you will have an imposing birch tree that will bring you pleasure from spring well into fall. Granted, the tannin-rich foliage will stay on the ground a long while and plug the gutters if the birch is too near the house—this tree's beauty and usefulness still will compensate you for this wrong. If you choose a silver birch (*Betula pendula*), you need not worry about its care or the soil in which it grows. Water it abundantly when you plant it in fall—that is all the care a birch needs. If you choose a sunny spot for it, it will show its gratitude through luxuriant growth.

The leaves are harvested in spring; dry them in the open air or in your kitchen oven at about 104°F (40°C). When freshly picked, the young leaves, minced, will also make a tasty, nourishing addition to springtime soups and stews, salads, or dishes prepared from soft cheese. Add the minced leaves to soups and stews shortly before serving.

Bitter Orange (Bigarade): Offers More Than Fragrance

The botanical name of the bitter orange, also known as the sour orange, Seville orange, or bigarade, is *Citrus aurantium, ssp. aurantium* or *ssp. amara*. It was bred specially for the extraction of pharmaceutical drugs, primarily in the West Indies and Spain. The bitter orange is only distantly related to the citrus fruits we eat—oranges, tangerines, and grapefruits.

The flowers, the small unripe fruits, and the peel—minus the white inner skin—are the parts used pharmaceutically. The flowers of the bitter orange have a pleasant scent; because they slightly subdue the nervous system, they are frequently added to calmative and sedative teas—

not only for the fragrance they contribute. The peel of the ripe fruits contains sweet-smelling essential oil with a great deal of limonene, as well as bitter-tasting flavonoids. Both these active substances are beneficial in treating lack of appetite and complete or partial failure to produce gastric juice. In addition, they promote digestion. Bitter-orange peel at one time was in common use as a medicament, but it unfortunately fell into obscurity. During the rebirth of natural medicines, the value of this healing agent was rediscovered. The German Office of Health recommends the bitter orange as a helpful medicinal plant to treat cases of insufficient production of gastric juice and to stimulate the appetite. Contraindications are listed as gastric and intestinal ulcers.

The bitter-orange tree is shallow-rooted. It grows up to almost 43 feet (13 m) tall and has a profusely branching, spherical crown. The leaves grow in a spiral pattern on the branches; the white flowers appear in the leaf axils. The flowers occasionally are also combined on the branches to form small flower stalks. From these

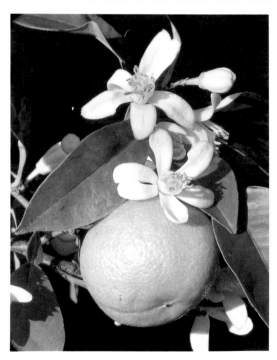

Bitter orange

flowers develop almost globular fruits, which resemble oranges in shape and appearance.

Cultivation

Growing bitter-orange trees is possible in the subtropical parts of North America. In more northerly latitudes, cultivate in pots that can be taken indoors during the winter. Bitter orange needs full sun. In a bright, subtropical location, it will bloom year round. In regions subject to frost, move indoors to a bright, airy location at 39 to 46°F (4–8°C). Water pots sparingly and provide good drainage. Move outdoors late in May.

Blackberry Leaves and Raspberry Leaves: Seemingly Made for House Teas

Rubus fruticosus L. is the botanical name of the blackberry; the raspberry is known to botanists as *Rubus idaeus* L. Both plants belong to the rose family (Rosaceae) and provide us with tasty fruits that, made into jam, stewed fruit, or juice, are as well known as they are well loved.

The leaves of these two vines are also put to use—as a tea for everyday consumption or as a basis for various tea blends for long-term use. If a doctor, for example, advises his patients with kidney problems to drink at least 2 quarts (2 L) of tea a day over a period of weeks and months, then the tea cannot be particularly strong, as the primary goal is the intake of large quantities of liquids to irrigate the urinary passages. A tea that consists of 50 percent raspberry and blackberry leaves and 50 percent diuretic tea herbs (for example, birch leaves, dandelion roots with the aerial parts, field horsetail, and the aerial parts of goldenrod) is particularly suitable for this purpose. Older people, who also need to drink plenty of liquids, can prepare tasty teas on a daily basis, using a tea blend of raspberry and blackberry leaves with the addition of peppermint or balm and rose hips or hibiscus.

Blackberry shrubs grow and proliferate in many different varieties and strains in flat coun-

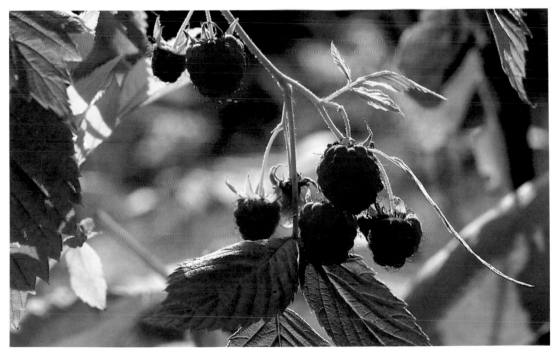

Raspberries

try as well as mountainous regions. They are found in landfills, thinly wooded areas, clearings, and completely deforested areas, and on embankments and sunny slopes. Their undergrowth can become virtually impenetrable, as the branches and twigs bear curved thorns. Blackberry shrubs have no single flowering season; they bloom from May well into winter, with pauses of varying lengths. For this reason, we find flowers, unripe fruits, and ripe fruits on the same shrub. The white to pale-reddish flowers produce blue-black berries in the form of syncarpous drupes, glossy in some species, pruinous in others. Some blackberries are fairly large, others relatively small; some taste aromatic, others watery. Pinnately divided blackberry leaves have five- to three-toothed leaflets, which are smooth on their upper side and hairy underneath. On the ribs of the leaves are small thorns.

Raspberry shrubs grow in the same habitats as blackberry shrubs. They reach a height of about 3 1/4 to 6 1/2 feet (1-2 m) and have leafy, often curved and slightly prickly canes with leaves in a palmate pattern, in which the small

terminal leaf is stalked. The small ovate leaves are covered with velvety hair underneath.

The color of raspberry flowers fluctuates between pure white and pale pink. The red fruits are syncarps, which can easily be lifted off the cone-shaped receptacles when they are ripe. The flowering season is in May and June (July); ripe fruits will be found into fall. The poorer the soil in which the shrub grows, the more fragrant the smell of the raspberries.

At one time raspberry juice, made from fully ripened berries, was frequently given to children with fever; it was increasingly replaced by juices of citrus fruits, although I don't see why. Raspberries also contain large amounts of vitamin C, along with B vitamins, provitamin A, and numerous minerals such as potassium, calcium, iron, magnesium, and microcosmic salts (sodium ammonium phosphate, or salt of phosphorus).

Cultivation

Even today, raspberries growing in your backyard garden, along the fence, or on trellises are still commonplace, at least in the countryside. As far as fruits and berries are concerned, cultivated raspberries are the equals of the wild forms; however, the blackberries that have been bred especially for garden owners have coarser leaves and larger fruits with a lower vitamin content. Nevertheless, giving a home to blackberries is recommended, provided your garden is large enough. It is inadvisable to bring wild blackberries into your garden, because they usually are quick to form an impenetrable, tangled thicket. Raspberry and blackberry shrubs are available in nurseries; the shrubs need a sunny location but can grow in any soil.

Black Currant: Much Used in Folk Medicine

Today the heading "black currant" immediately calls to mind the juice of the ripe berries, which is quite rich in vitamins and minerals. The vitamin C content of the ripe berries, 120 milligrams

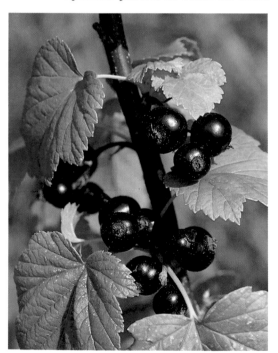

Black currant

per 3.52 ounces (100 g), is said to far exceed that of citrus fruits. Vitamins of the B complex, and other vitamins are also present in black currants. The raw berries, the juice pressed from the ripe berries, black currant jam, or stewed black currants are healthful for children and adults. Far less well-known is the use of a tea made from the dried black currant leaves. In folk medicine, this tea has been used for many decades to treat rheumatism and gout. Bouts of rheumatic pain become less frequent and less severe after a course of treatment (drink two cups of tea daily for four to six weeks). Nevertheless, orthodox medicine is quite reserved, and the German Office of Health grants the tea made from black currant leaves only a mild diuretic effect.

Ribes nigrum L. is the botanical name of the black currant, which belongs to the gooseberry family (Grossulariaceae). In central and eastern Europe it grows wild and is known under a variety of common names—for example, "goutberry."

The leaves have three to five lobes and are coarsely serrate. Oil glands appear on the undersides of the leaves. The flowers, which grow in hanging racemes, or clusters, are yellowish-green, with brownish-red margins. From the flowers develop berries that at first are brownish-red, then turn deep black. The entire plant has an odor that ranges from pungent to unpleasant, which explains some of its common names: stinkshrub, bugberry, and stallberry. This odor largely disappears when the fruits are processed and the leaves are dried. If you would like to harvest black currant leaves in your own garden, make sure you pick only healthy, "clean" berries, because black currant bushes often are infested with a fungus (the crown rust typical of this plant).

Cultivation

"One of every three currant bushes in your garden should be a black currant, as 1:2 is also the right mixing ratio for making a nourishing jam." I found this information in an old book of home remedies, and I share the belief that black currants belong in every sizable backyard garden.

The bushes are easy to grow, as they require no care apart from an annual cutting back.

The bushes are available in larger garden centers, where you also can get advice on fertilizing and cutting back.

Blueberry: The Leaves and the Fruits Are Equally Desirable

Blueberries, also commonly known as bilberries, huckleberries, hurtleberries, or whortleberries, will turn your mouth, lips, and tongue a lovely shade of blue. These fruits of *Vaccinium myrtillus* L., a member of the heath family (Ericaceae), continue to be gathered eagerly; they are eaten raw with sugar or milk or made into jam, jelly, or wine.

Dried blueberries, however, are a time-tested remedy for various types of diarrhea, as scientists acknowledge. The German Office of Health makes this recommendation: To assist in the treatment of acute and specific diarrheal disorders.

In folk medicine, a tea made from dried blueberries is commonly used to combat "teething diarrhea" in small children. Blueberry tea made from the dried fruits also is a good gargle and mouthwash for those suffering from inflamed oral mucosae.

Please note

I do not recommend the widespread use of blueberry leaves, still quite popular in folk medicine. First, there is no evidence of its effectiveness against diabetes, bladder and kidney catarrhs, rheumatism, and heart trouble; second, if the application is continued for a long time, the leaves can induce chronic poisoning (by hydroquinone). Therefore: Don't use blueberry-leaf tea!

Vaccinium myrtillus, the blueberry bush, is a small subshrub that can reach a height of about 20 inches (50 cm). It is commonly found in shady woods, in peat bogs, and on stretches of heath, where it forms extensive colonies. Its green stems are squared and profusely branched. The firm leaves, which grow on very short

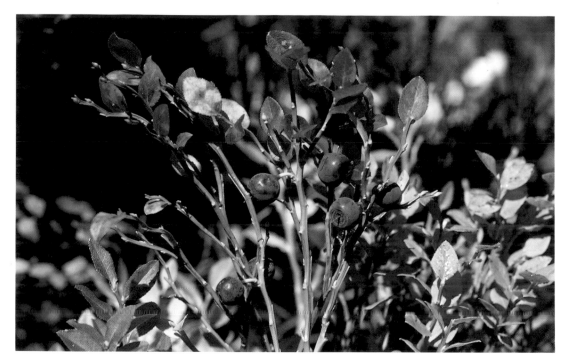

Blueberries

stalks, are ovate, slightly serrate along the margin, and alternate. In their axils grow, singly or in pairs, the bell-shaped, spherical green flowers flushed with red, which produce blue-black berries in summer. The deep blue juice distinguishes the blueberry from the bog bilberry (*Vaccinium uliginosum*), which produces egg-shaped berries with greenish-brown juice.

Cultivation
Wild blueberries and their cultivars can be purchased from local nurseries.

Caraway: One of the Oldest Medicinal Plants

The famous Ebers Papyrus, an 80-foot (20 m) ancient Egyptian scroll containing medical notes and recipes from 1550 B.C., lists 20 plants used as both medicines and seasonings, including anise, fennel, thyme, mustard, wormwood, and caraway. Thus we know that caraway has been in use for at least 3500 years.

Today we prize caraway equally as a flavoring and as a medicinal tea. The tea relieves gas pains and the sensation of fullness that follows the eating of hard-to-digest foods. In Bavaria caraway is added, for example, to every pork roast as a seasoning. The medicinal effect of caraway is due principally to the carvon contained in the essential oil.

The German Office of Health endorses the use of caraway as a medicinal tea for relief of the aforementioned complaints and also names other areas of application: mild cramplike gastrointestinal complaints and nervous cardiac and circulatory conditions.

Carum carvi L., as botanists call caraway, belongs to the carrot family (Apiaceae = Umbelliferae). This family also includes anise, fennel, and coriander, which are similar in effect.

The stem of this approximately 39-inch (1 m) medicinal plant is profusely branched, squared, and ungrooved. It bears four-part leaves in pairs.

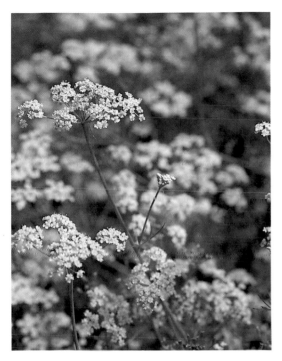

Caraway

Caraway is a biennial that is raised from seed (available at seed stores). Sow it in March and April, in rows about 12 inches (30 cm) apart, and press the seeds lightly into the soil. After about two weeks you can see the first seedlings, which in the first year develop into leaf rosettes. After several weeks thin out the rows, leaving enough vigorous plants for your needs—they have to be at least 8 inches (20 cm) apart to permit continued vigorous growth. In the second year the leaf rosette will send forth the flowering and fruiting shoots, and in June or July the caraway fruits (seeds) will be ripe. After the harvest, dry the ripe seeds again in your oven and store them in a screw-top jar made of opaque glass.

Occasionally these leaves are red. The umbels have seven to ten main rays.

Caraway is indigenous to Eurasia, where it is often seen in meadows, pastures, and grassy areas and along slopes and embankments. Nevertheless, the caraway used as a seasoning and a medicine comes almost exclusively from cultivation.

Please note
Caraway belongs to the carrot family, which includes a great many poisonous species that can easily be mistaken for this plant. For this reason, do not collect wild caraway under any circumstances!

Cultivation
To meet your own needs, you should have at least ten specimens of this plant, which is about 39 inches (1 m) tall when mature. This means that you can grow caraway only in a large garden. It needs slightly loamy, nutritious soil (ask at a garden store) and a sunny location in your garden, because it germinates in the light.

Celandine: An Antispasmodic for the Gastrointestinal Region

This plant has been used in medicine for an extremely long time. In the writings of the Greek philosopher Theophrastus (372–287 B.C.), we read that celandine is useful in treating jaundice, liver disease, constipation, and gallstones. These findings also entered into the medieval herbals, from which folk medicine draws its knowledge. Nevertheless, it is necessary to point out that celandine tea by itself is seldom used any more. Instead, celandine is an active ingredient of teas for the stomach, intestinal tract, gallbladder, and liver. It also is used in Galenic preparations in the form of drops. I consider tea blends containing celandine quite appropriate, owing to its antispasmodic effect.

Botanists call this medicinal plant *Chelidonium majus* and assign it to the poppy family (Papaveraceae). Introduced in this country from Europe, the plant now grows principally along walls, paths, and fences and in landfills. Occasionally it grows right out of a high old wall, into the cracks of which ants have carried the seeds, because celandine seeds have an appendage that ants find delicious.

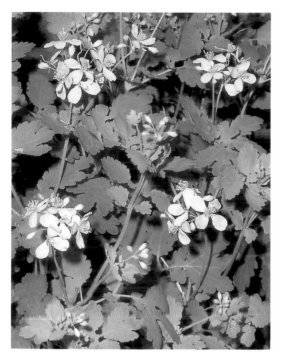

Celandine

Chelidonium, a perennial, is anchored in the soil with a strong root. Depending on the habitat, it grows from 12 inches (30 cm) to over 39 inches (1 m) tall. All its parts contain a yellowish milky juice with which people try to get rid of warts and pimples. Celandine stems are branching, slightly hairy, and covered with hairy alternate leaves. The leaves are bluish-green, pinnatifid at the top and pinnate at the bottom. The bright-yellow flowers have four petals and numerous stamens. The fruit, which bursts open (dehisces) by means of two valves, contains black seeds with a white appendage. Celandine blooms from March to the end of November; the primary blooming season is during the months of May and June.

The German Office of Health acknowledges the efficacy of celandine in the treatment of cramplike disturbances in the area of the bile ducts and the gastrointestinal tract.

Cultivation

Celandine is not highly recommended for raising in your backyard garden. If it finds its own way in, however, and turns up along fences or old garden walls, then you ought to grant it asylum. Because it is a perennial, you can count on its reappearance every year.

Chamomile: Valued for Centuries

Botanists now call it *Chamomilla recutita*, although the designations *Matricaria chamomilla* and *Matricaria recutita* are still in use as well.

Chamomile has been known to folk medicine for many centuries; it is among the most extensively studied medicinal plants. The German Office of Health also expressly acknowledges the beneficial effect of chamomile in allaying gastric and intestinal conditions.

For medicinal purposes, the parts used are the dried flower heads.

The most important component of this medicinal plant is the essential oil, containing up to 50 percent alpha-bisabolol as well as chamazulene, a blue substance. The unique healing effect of chamomile results from the joint action of all the substances it contains.

Chamomile tea is used for stomach and intestinal conditions and also for states of restlessness. Other preparations such as drops, ointments, and healing cosmetic products also are made from chamomile. This medicinal plant is effective wherever there is a need to ease soreness and swelling.

Chamomile is an undemanding plant that grows in fields and landfills, on fallow land, and along roadsides, embankments, and field boundaries. It once was a common weed in grain fields, but since the introduction of herbicides its numbers have been greatly reduced.

From a short root chamomile puts forth a stem 8 to 20 inches (20–50 cm) tall, from which bi- to tripinnatipartite leaves grow. The small flower heads, which grow singly at the ends of the shoot tips, consist of a corona of white

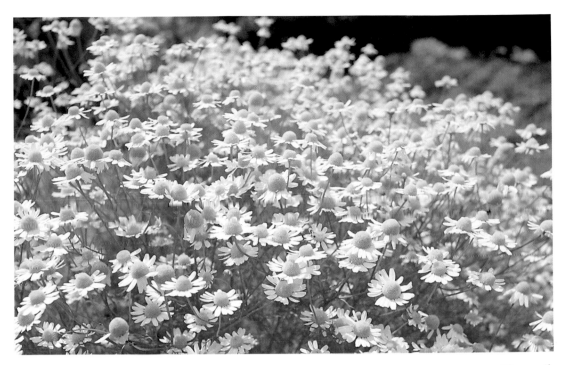

Chamomile

ligulate flowers and many (up to 400) yellow tubular disk flowers at the center. They bloom from May to June. The fruits (seeds) are extremely tiny: About 20,000 of them weigh .035 ounce (1 g).

There are other species called chamomile. Cases of mistaken identity may result in allergic reactions to the application of chamomile. Consequently, buy chamomile in a pharmacy or health food store.

Cultivation

Growing chamomile in your garden or in bowls and pots on your balcony or patio is quite rewarding, because once the "chamomile culture" is established, you need not tend it. The seeds cast by this annual will produce plenty of new plants each year. However, chamomile does need humus, nutritious soil that is not too heavy and plenty of sun. If there is no rainfall for a prolonged period you will have to water (ask at a garden store).

Chamomile seeds are sold in every seed store. Sow them in spring in well-prepared (loosened) soil, which has to be kept damp at first. Because chamomile germinates in the light, all you need to do is to broadcast the seeds and press them down very lightly.

Chamomile grows 8 to 20 inches (20–50 cm) tall and blooms from May to June. Harvest the flower heads as soon as they have opened, taking as little of the stalk as possible.

Comfrey: Only for External Use

Comfrey is an extremely old medicinal plant with an amazing effect. Even Abbess Hildegard of Bingen praised it as an external application for broken bones, and Paracelsus also sang comfrey's praises. Suppurating and poorly healing wounds are improved rapidly by application of a comfrey compress, which also can accelerate the healing of hematomas, swellings, and ulcerated

Branching stems that grow 20 to 39 inches (50–100 cm) tall rise from a thick rhizome that is black outside, white and juicy inside. On the stems grow lanceolate leaves, hairy and rough, narrowing at the petiole. The purplish, occasionally also yellowish-white flowers are bell-shaped and bloom in drooping clusters, or racemes, from May to September.

Cultivation

Buy several plants from a garden center and set them at least 12 inches (30 cm) apart in humus-rich garden soil. Partially shady or shady locations are suitable. Frequent watering in case of dryness is all the care they need; the plants will grow vigorously and propagate on their own, without further ado.

Common or Field Horsetail: Also Known as Scouring Rush

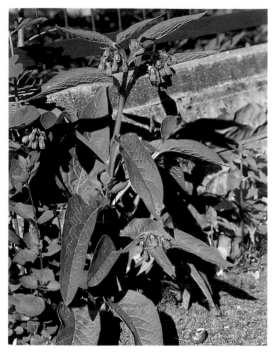

Comfrey

legs (varicose ulcers). All these properties were known many, many years ago.

The German Office of Health, however, is quite reserved in its assessment of this medicinal plant, because comfrey root—the part used for medicinal purposes—contains minute quantities of toxic pyrrolizidine alkaloids in addition to the important active substance allantoin, responsible for its healing properties.

Please note

Internal application—in the form of comfrey tea—is not advisable.

Comfrey's botanical name is *Symphytum officinale* L.; it belongs to the borage family (Boraginaceae). It also has numerous common names, including ass-ear, blackwort, bruisewort, healing herb, knitback, knitbone, and consolida.

Comfrey is common in this country as an escaped introduced plant from Europe. It prefers wet places along streams and rivers. It grows in damp meadows as well as along roadsides and in fields and underbrush.

The medicinally useful parts of common or field horsetail (*Equisetum arvense*) (Equisetaceae or horsetail family), are not the structures shown in the photo, the fertile spore-bearing shoots that sprout from the soil in February and March, but the sterile summer shoots that appear later, the horsetail. When dried in the open air and cut into small pieces suitable for making tea, they yield horsetail tea.

The use of common or field horsetail can be traced to antiquity, for "hippuris" (the Greek word for horsetail, on account of the appearance of the sterile shoots), mentioned by Dioscorides (about A.D. 50), was a favorite diuretic and styptic agent even then. Albertus Magnus (1193-1280) shared this opinion, and in more recent times Sebastian Kneipp also praised horsetail for its power to stop bleeding, calling it "peerless, irreplaceable." It is now an important remedy in folk medicine—a "blood purifier" in spring and fall, a means of treating rheumatism and gout, and a cough and asthma remedy. It also is used to alleviate accumulations of water in the body (edema) and to treat skin blemishes, brittle fingernails, and damaged hair. In the face of so

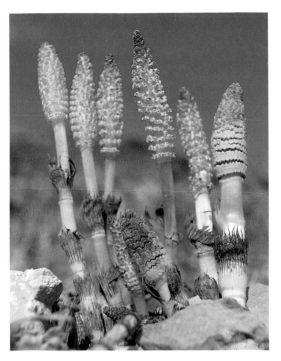

Common or Field horsetail

Cultivation
If you wish, you may of course put common or field horsetail in your garden, as this medicinal plant is satisfied with almost any soil. It prefers, as its name suggests, average plowland, or soil from a field, and if it is slightly loamy, the horsetail will be especially content. Because this plant is a common field weed, you can simply dig up a bushy specimen at the edge of a country road—assuming that you can identify the plant with certainty! Set it in a sunny spot in your garden. Nothing more is necessary. You will first begin to enjoy this medicinal plant in spring, when the spore-bearing shoots sprout from the ground. The multibranched bushy stems of common or field horsetail that sprout in summer and are used to make tea are less attractive; incidentally, they also are good for scouring old pewter.

much eulogizing and general approval, a question naturally arises: What do we really think of this medicinal plant today? Scientists, who apply very strict standards, are reserved in their judgment; the German Office of Health offers the following recommendation: "Horsetail tea promotes the flow of urine and is also used for supplementary treatment of catarrhs in the kidney and bladder areas." This means that horsetail (like goldenrod, stinging nettle, and dandelion) always can be employed successfully if the doctor, in treating bladder and kidney problems, advises the patient to drink plenty of liquids.

The aerial parts of horsetail are also components of many tea blends used to treat rheumatism, gout, coughs, and colds.

With most diuretic teas, the German Office of Health points out that they are contraindicated if the retention of water in the body is due to cardiac or renal insufficiency (impaired performance). It is up to the doctor to determine whether that is the case.

Coriander: Medicinal Plant and Kitchen Herb

Coriandrum sativum L. is the botanical name of this medicinal plant and kitchen herb, a member of the carrot family (Apiaceae = Umbelliferae).

Coriander also is known as Chinese parsley or cilantro. Among its common names are bugbane, bug dill, and stinking dill, because the seeds (fruits), if harvested while unripe, will retain an unpleasant odor even after they have been dried. Only coriander seeds harvested after they are fully ripe have a pleasantly spicy smell, slightly reminiscent of the fragrance of lilies of the valley.

For medicinal purposes, the parts used are the ripe coriander seeds. They contain essential oils that are effective remedies for flatulence and the sensation of fullness, as well as for cramplike pain in the gastrointestinal area. Coriander is

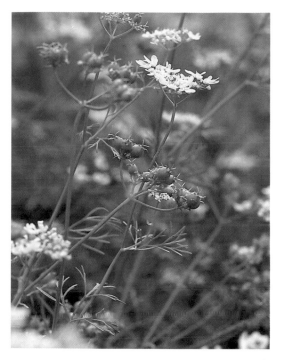

Coriander

The globular fruits never fall apart into their mericarps, as is otherwise the case with the dehiscent fruits of the Umbelliferae.

> **Please note**
> Coriander belongs to the carrot family, which includes many poisonous species that may be mistaken for this medicinal plant!

Cultivation

Raising coriander in your backyard garden is not advisable in the northernmost parts of the United States and Canada because the climate is too harsh for this plant, and consequently the seeds (fruits) are unable to ripen fully. In more temperate areas, sow in the spring. Caution is required to transplant the seedlings, which should be spaced about 3 inches (7.5 cm) apart. Grow in full sun or partial shade. Leaves (for use as a seasoning) may be picked from the tops of plants 6 inches (15 cm) or more high. Seeds may be collected when fully ripe—usually in the late summer.

especially suitable for treatment of gas in the epigastric region. The German Office of Health also recommends coriander for supportive treatment of epigastric conditions such as a feeling of fullness, flatulence, and mild cramplike stomach and intestinal upsets.

Coriander has been used for 3000 years as a seasoning; coriander seeds were found in Egyptian tombs dating from about 1000 B.C. In Germany, bread is frequently flavored with coriander, and it also is an ingredient of curry powder.

Coriander is thought to have originated in the eastern Mediterranean region and the Near East. From there it crossed the Alps to monastery gardens and later found its way into farmers' gardens.

The plant reaches a height of about 20 inches (50 cm). It has bare, round stems, which branch in the plant's upper part. The lower leaves are long-stemmed, sometimes entire or simply pinnatisect. The higher the leaves are on the plant, the more divided are the leaf blades and the shorter are the petioles. The small white or slightly reddish flowers grow in double umbels with three to five rays.

Couch Grass (Quack Grass): An Effective Acne Remedy

Couch grass, *Elymus repens*, also known as *Agropyron repens*, is a widespread weed in the Northern Hemisphere. It belongs to the grass family (Poaceae = Gramineae). For medicinal purposes, the part used is the dried rhizome (*Graminis rhizoma*), which contains triticin—a polysaccharide (carbohydrate) similar to the inulin found in dandelion—mucilage, sugar, and silicic acid. This drug was already in use in olden times: as a tonic, a dietary food for diabetics, a specific for rheumatism and gout, and, above all, as a remedy for chronic skin eruptions. Couch grass roots also were valued as a cough remedy. Scientists, however, are extremely reserved in recommending this drug. In the package circular stipulated by the German Office of Health, it says only this: To increase urine flow in catarrhs of the urinary passages; as an adjunct to the treatment of catarrhs of the upper respiratory passages.

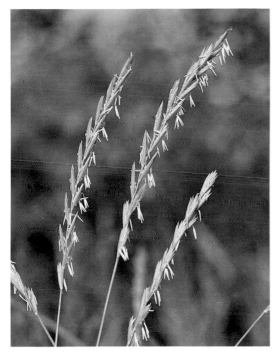

Couch Grass (Quack Grass)

(55°C) to prevent mold formation. The dried roots will keep for several years if protected from dampness.

Cultivation
Growing couch grass in your backyard garden is inadvisable, because it proliferates so profusely that it is hard to eradicate.

Dandelion: Highly Esteemed as a Medicinal Plant

This medicinal plant, esteemed primarily in folk medicine, is at home throughout the entire Northern Hemisphere. Its great adaptability and its ability to be content with little are admirable. Wherever the wind blows the seeds, equipped with their well-known "parachutes," they find a foothold. Dandelion grows and blooms in cracks in concrete, in parking lots, between paving stones downtown, and on old walls, as well as in meadows and fields and along roadsides.

A tea, however, has proved helpful, particularly with acne and other skin diseases. It is drunk as a beverage or used externally as a wash. Couch grass root finds support in pansies (see page 193) and the aerial parts of eyebright (see page 166). Stinging nettle leaves (see page 120) and the aerial parts of field horsetail (see page 154) also complement the effect of couch grass root.

Elymus repens, or couch grass, is anchored in the ground with a rhizome that becomes extremely long as it creeps and produces a great many stolons. This makes the grass practically impossible to eradicate; wherever it becomes established, it reproduces with incredible speed. From the rhizome an erect, bare stem rises to the surface; it bears narrow, green or bluish-green flat leaves and reaches a height of more than 39 inches (1 m). Atop each stem is a flower spike. The blooming period is June to August.

Couch grass roots are harvested in spring before new stems form from the rhizome. Wash the roots and dry them first in the open air, then with artificial heat at a temperature of 131°F

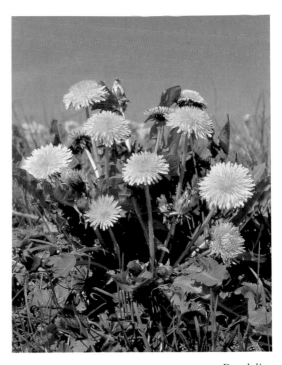

Dandelion

Depending on the properties of the soil, it grows sometimes luxuriant and large, sometimes delicate and small. Anchored in the ground with a powerful taproot, it produces a basal rosette with irregularly toothed leaves that hold a white milky juice. From the center of this leaf rosette develops the inflorescence, shaped like a tiny basket and located at the end of a hollow stem that also contains milky juice.

The dandelion, known to botanists as *Taraxacum officinale*, belongs to the composite family (Asteraceae = Compositae). The golden-yellow inflorescences show their dazzling color in early spring; dandelion starts to bloom as early as March. After flowering has ceased, the yellow blossoms turn into silvery white balls of fruits, the "puffs," with seeds that have parachutelike appendages.

It is not surprising that such a handsome, unusual plant attracted people's attention long ago. In spring, the leaves were eaten as salad greens to compensate for the lack of vitamins and minerals during the cold winter months. Dandelion was also used as a spring tonic. Not least, its diuretic properties and ability to stimulate the kidneys and bladder were put to use in a medicinal tea.

People with rheumatism tried the tea and found it soothing. Those with gallbladder and liver conditions were also satisfied with its effect, and anyone troubled with skin blemishes used dandelion tea or dandelion juice in a course of treatment.

And today? The popularity of the dandelion remains virtually unchanged, but because it lacks distinctive active substances, scientists are quite conservative in their assessment. The recommendation of the German Office of Health is as follows: Disturbances in the gastrointestinal area such as a sensation of fullness, flatulence, and indigestion.

In this endorsement the diuretic effect of dandelion tea has been overlooked, as has its potential for use to expel kidney or bladder stones and renal gravel with a massive dose of water or to exert a beneficial influence on arthrosis (joint diseases). Indeed, it has anti-inflammatory activity, which has recently been confirmed in animal studies.

I would like to encourage everyone to do the following: As often as possible, but particularly in spring, eat a salad of dandelion greens, mix finely chopped dandelion leaves with farmer's cheese or some other soft cheese, and add chopped dandelion leaves to soups and stews shortly before serving. Your stomach, intestines, gallbladder, liver, bladder, and kidneys will thank you for doing so.

Cultivation

If you own an orchard, dandelion will be a permanent guest. Every spring it will be back, usually in huge numbers—once it strikes root somewhere, there it stays. It is undemanding in terms of the soil in which it grows, and its ability to adapt is astonishing.

For medicinal purposes the parts used are the roots and leaves, which are employed as a drug for dandelion tea and numerous tea blends.

The roots and leaves are harvested in spring before the blooming season. Because the root reaches deep into the ground, you need a root-digging tool for harvesting. Wash the leaves and roots briefly, cut them into small pieces, and dry them in your oven, with its door open, at a temperature of about 122°F (50°C) (see page 138).

Dill: At Its Best when Fresh

You should put dill in your backyard garden, not least in order to have fresh dill available when you want it. Botanists call it *Anethum graveolens*, and its popularity corresponds to that of some of its relatives in the carrot family (Apiaceae = Umbelliferae): caraway, anise, fennel, and coriander.

Dill has been known to us for several thousand years. The Egyptians prized it as highly as did the Greeks and Romans, principally as a culinary herb, but one of medicinal benefit, because its presence as a seasoning often is sufficient to prevent flatulence and a feeling of fullness. Dill, it is said, is a native of the Orient, but today it is found in cultures and gardens

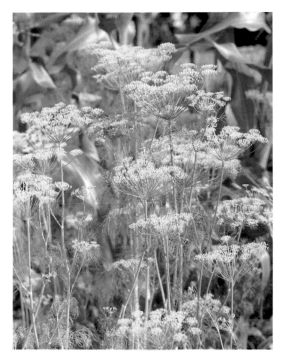

Dill

teaspoonful of minced dill weed and blend the mixture with a mortar and pestle or rub it against a grater. This mixture, spread on toast, has a delicious taste.

Please note
Dill belongs to the carrot family, which includes a host of poisonous species that may be mistaken for this medicinal plant!

Cultivation
Dill is grown as an annual from seed sown in April at intervals of two to three weeks, to ensure that fresh dill weed can be harvested over a long period of time. Plant the rows 10 inches (25 cm) apart, to allow the plants to develop fully. Dill needs light to germinate. It should be sown at a shallow depth and pressed down very lightly. Dill likes heavy, loamy soil but cannot tolerate standing water.

For household use, harvest the fresh dill weed as needed. For pickling and preserving, harvest the entire plant during the blooming period; dry it in bunches in the open air.

throughout Europe and all the Americas, as well as South Africa and East Africa.

Dill is a relatively undemanding annual, an umbelliferous plant that can reach a height of over 39 inches (1 m). Its finely grooved hollow stem, which is covered with a bluish frostlike bloom, bears thin pinnatisect foliage leaves. The upper leaves are less profusely articulated than the lower stem leaves. They terminate in extremely fine, long, filamentous leaf lobes, which are sold under the name of dill weed. They also have the finest aroma and, as the saying goes, the ability to make fresh foods taste even fresher. The taste of cucumbers, fish, soups, sauces, salads, and egg dishes is improved and refined by fresh dill. Dill leaves are also quite popular for seasoning pickled and preserved foods. Age-old experience teaches us that dill weed, if added in large amounts to salads, soups, and stews, will increase milk production in nursing women. The following recipe is especially recommended:

With a fork, mash two soft-boiled eggs fine and add a pinch of salt. To this, add 1 heaping

Elderberry: Flowers and Fruit are Beautiful and Useful

Even such well-known medicinal plants as peppermint, lemon balm, or chamomile have a hard time competing with the popularity of the elderberry, or elder. The ancient Germans believed it to be the dwelling place of Mother Hulda, the protectress of house and home. On virtually every German farm property an elderberry shrub could be found near the house or the stalls or, even more commonly, in the garden. There is legitimate reason to assume that elderberry was used for medicinal purposes even in prehistoric times.

Metabolic diseases like rheumatism and gout are treated with elderberry flower tea, and it also is used to activate the body's powers of resistance and even to treat skin blemishes. These usages, however—including drinking the tea to

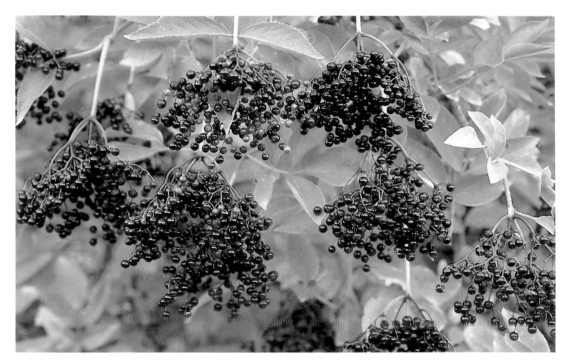

Elderberry

alleviate cold symptoms—lie within the realm of folk medicine. Orthodox science is more reserved, because thus far no "particular active substances" have been found that can explain all these applications.

The German Office of Health recommends elderberry flowers as a diaphoretic in the treatment of colds accompanied by fever.

Botanists call elderberry *Sambucus nigra* and assign it to the honeysuckle family (Caprifoliaceae). It is common in hedges and thickets and along roads and the banks of streams. Elderberry is a shrub or small tree that branches profusely and can grow up to approximately 10 to 23 feet (3–7 m) tall. Important features are its warty, unpleasant-smelling bark, pithy limbs and branches, and opposite, imparipinnate leaves. Other unmistakable characteristics of the black elderberry are the large, shallow, false umbelliferous inflorescences with small yellowish-white flowers that bloom in May and June, and the blue-black berries that ripen in fall and grow in hanging clusters.

Cultivation

In the countryside, in farmers' gardens, and next to barns and stalls, the elderberry is an essential part of the picture. Go ahead and put it in your garden too. In spring it is an adornment and provides us with medicinally useful flowers; in fall it yields the black fruits that you can make into stewed fruit, jam, juice, or even wine or liqueur.

Nothing is easier than planting and tending an elderberry in your garden. Get a small shrub from a nursery, set it in humus soil, water it well, and leave the rest to this rapidly growing shrub itself. It prefers partial shade but can put up with stronger sun, provided you water it occasionally in periods of scant rainfall. And it won't die in the shade, either.

In May and June, elderberry will delight you with masses of yellowish-white flowers arranged in false umbelliferous inflorescences. It is the flowers that are used for medicinal purposes. Harvest them by cutting off the inflorescences whole and drying them in the open air, where you later can strip off the tiny flowers. Store them in containers that can be tightly closed to protect them from light and humidity, so that the tea will retain its effectiveness. Damp flowers get musty and lose both aroma and effect.

In fall, harvest the completely ripe berries—they are not poisonous, as is frequently assumed—and make them into jam, stewed fruit, or tasty elderberry soups. Plenty of recipes are available.

English Plantain: Its Leaves Help to Ease Coughs

Plantago lanceolata is the botanical name of English plantain. If you are familiar with it, you will encounter it at every turn, for it grows everywhere—in dry meadows, fields, and landfills and along the roadside. There are two closely related species, which are to be found in the same places: common plantain (*Plantago major*), with broad, oval leaves and a long inflorescence on a shorter stalk, and hoary plantain (*Plantago media*), which occupies an inter-mediate position in terms of its leaves and inflorescence. The leaves of all three species are used for medicinal purposes.

In both folk medicine and orthodox medicine, English plantain is recognized as a cough remedy. It is an ingredient of many tea blends and is also used in the form of a fresh juice.

The German Office of Health acknowledges English plantain as effective in the treatment of catarrhs of the upper respiratory passages. Mucilage, bitter constituents, silicic acid and the glucoside aucubin, flavonoids, numerous minerals, and tannins are probably to be viewed as active substances.

The English plantain commonly grows wild as a naturalized introduced plant.

English plantain is a perennial that is anchored in the ground with a strong rhizome. The leaves grow in a basal rosette. They reach a length of 8 to 16 inches (20–40 cm) and are narrow to lanceolate and only slightly hairy, with distinct longitudinal veins. Three to seven leaf veins are apparent. From the center of this leaf rosette arise erect leafless stalks 4 to 16 inches (10–40 cm) long, each of which bears at its tip a rather short, cylindrical to spherical flower spike with small flowers. The flowers produce fine, delicate stamens, which during the blooming season rise high above the tiny flowers. English plantain blooms from May to September; during this time the flowers, which are used for pharmaceutical purposes, can be gathered, then dried in the open air (see page 140).

In conclusion, one more application drawn from folk medicine, one I consider worth recommending: If you have been stung by insects and immediately rub some crushed English plantain leaves into the area around the sites of the stings, you will prevent swelling and itching.

Cultivation
English plantain is not well suited for raising in your own herb garden. Moreover, it is so common in the wild that you will easily find plenty of leaves for your household medicine chest of herbs.

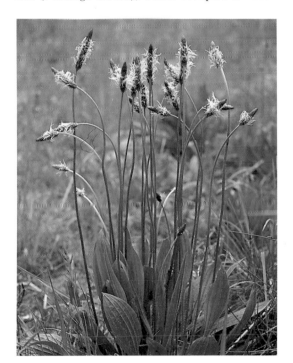

English Plantain

Erect Cinquefoil: A Reliable Remedy for Diarrhea

Erect cinquefoil, also known as bloodroot, tormentil, or tormentilla, has the botanical name of *Potentilla erecta* and belongs to the rose family (Rosaceae). "Dysentery root," one of its German common names, indicates that the plant has long been valued as a remedy for diarrhea.

Erect cinquefoil has a wide range; it is found in Europe, Asia, North Africa, and North America. It grows on slopes and embankments, in heathland and in clearings, in sandy soil and in damp, marshy ground—although it does need sunlight and warmth.

For pharmaceutical purposes, the part used is the rhizome, which by virtue of its high tannin content is a good remedy for diarrhea. This is also confirmed by the German Office of Health, with this recommendation: For acute nonspecific diarrhea. Reference is also made to the fact that stomach irritations and vomiting may occasionally appear in sensitive patients. Also popular and extremely effective is a tea made from erect cinquefoil used as a gargle in treating inflammations in the mouth and throat areas.

Erect cinquefoil reaches a height of 4 to 16 inches (10–40 cm). Several forked branches, which bear feathery leaves, grow from a coarse, irregularly thick rhizome. At the end of each forked branch grows a yellow flower with four petals. The plants bloom from March to May.

A medieval legend tells how mankind came by this medicinal plant: In 1348–1349 the plague was raging in the town of Wiesental in Baden. When the crisis was at its worst and salvation seemed impossible, a bird came out of the heavens and allegedly sang this song, so distinctly that everyone could understand: "Eat tormentil (erect cinquefoil) and pimpernel (burnet), then you'll get well."

Cultivation

Raising erect cinquefoil yourself is not recommended.

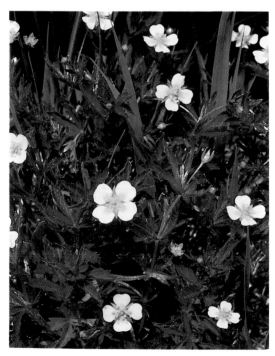

Erect Cinquefoil

Eucalyptus: The Oil Is Used to Treat Coughs and Colds

The eucalyptus tree, which is native to southwestern Australia and Tasmania, now grows in southern California and in many other regions as well.

The eucalyptus tree, *Eucalyptus globulus*, belongs to the myrtle family (Myrtaceae). Because it grows rapidly, it is used in Africa to drain malarial swamps. The common name given it there—fever tree—indicates that through its help in draining the swamps, the breeding grounds of the malarial (anopheles) mosquito are being eliminated and hence the fever—that is, malaria—is becoming less common.

The eucalyptus grows up to almost 230 feet (70 m) tall. It has gray-white bark. On young trees or new branches of older trees grow opposite, thin, ovate leaves, whereas the mature types of leaves are alternate, twice as thick, leathery, and much longer, with petioles. The principal

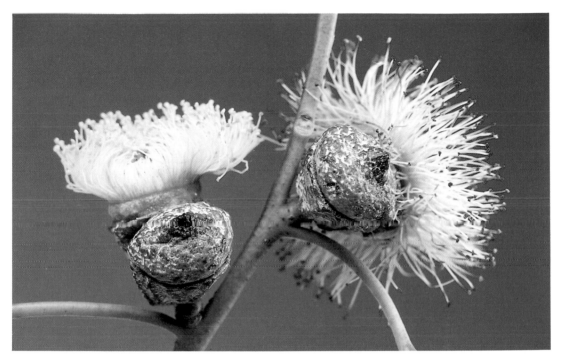

Eucalyptus

vein is quite prominent on the blue-green underside of the leaf, and it branches at a right angle. The secondary veins join to form an unforked marginal vein (craspedromus) that runs parallel to the leaf margin. The white eucalyptus flowers develop into coarse fruits.

The parts used for medicinal purposes are the leaves, which now are used only rarely as an ingredient of teas for colds. They are, however, used to produce the sought-after eucalyptus oil by means of steam distillation. Good leaves for commercial use should contain about 3 percent essential oil. Eucalyptus oil contains about 80 percent cineol (= eucalyptol). This oil is responsible for the pleasant effect in treatment of colds, as it is antiseptic, mucolytic, and refrigerant.

The number of ready-made preparations that contain eucalyptus oil is enormous. Every kind of product is represented, from pure oil through oil-containing ointments and rubs to candies and syrups. The effect is convincing, and side effects from the tea or from any of the commercial preparations are extremely rare.

Please note

With an overdose (this applies to all essential oils), nausea, vomiting, and diarrhea have been observed. Very few people have developed an allergy to eucalyptus oil.

Cultivation

In our latitudes, except California, the Southwest, and parts of Florida, it is impossible to grow eucalyptus trees yourself.

European Alder-Buckthorn: Reliable in Its Effect

Rhamnus frangula is the botanical name of European alder-buckthorn, also known by the common names of buckthorn, black dogwood, arrowwood, and glossy buckthorn.

The part used for medicinal purposes is the bark, harvested in spring. After it is stored for one year, the bark is a well-tested, drastic laxative. European alder-buckthorn bark is an

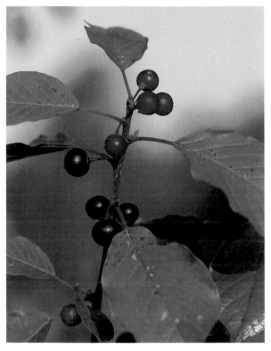

European Alder-Buckthorn

Cultivation
Raising European alder-buckthorn yourself is not recommended; the flowers are inconspicuous, the berries, poisonous.

European Centaury: The Bitter Medicine

Botanists know this member of the gentian family (Gentianaceae) as *Centaurium erythraea*. This medicinal plant has many common names, including forking centaury, bitter herb, bluebottle, bluet, feverwort, red centaury, and Christ's ladder.

anthraquinone drug, which in its effect is fully the equal of senna leaves and cascara bark. My recommendations concerning the use of senna (see page 203) also apply to European alder-buckthorn bark.

European alder-buckthorn is a deciduous shrub or small tree that belongs to the buckthorn family (Rhamnaceae). It grows up to almost 20 feet (6 m) tall and is common in Europe, growing in lowland forests and in marshy regions covered with alders, along roadsides, and in hedgerows. European alder-buckthorn is conspicuous because of the numerous gray lenticels (bodies of cells that serve as pores) on its otherwise smooth, gray-brown, glossy bark. The modest white flowers grow at the joints of the elliptical, entire-margined, glossy foliage leaves, which are arranged in an alternate pattern on the branches. From the fertilized flowers develop stone fruits, or drupes, green at first, then turning red and, when ripe, blue-violet to blue-black.

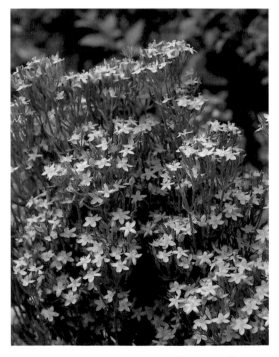

European Centaury

European centaury is a pure bitter-constituent plant that has been used since time immemorial as a tonic, a remedy for poor digestion and lack of appetite. It is still used in the same ways today. A saying from earlier times, when "bitter" was still a synonym for "efficacious," goes like this: "Medicine has to taste bitter; otherwise, it won't do any good."

The bitter constituents, mainly mixtures of secoiridoid glycosides and a few alkaloids, are the only active ingredients of interest in European centaury; they are responsible for improving the flow of peptic juice throughout the digestive tract, which results in an improved appetite, trouble-free assimilation of food, and a state of well-being. The recommendation of the German Office of Health is as follows: To promote the production of peptic juice (gastritis with insufficient production of peptic acid), and as an appetite stimulant.

European centaury grows in Europe, Asia, North Africa, and North America. In Germany it is found in damp meadows and in thinly wooded areas. The stem is four-cornered and grows to a height of 4 to 20 inches (10 50 cm). The leaves are decussate. The red, star-shaped flowers, which open only when the sun shines, are arranged in umbellike panicles.

Please note

Do not collect this medicinal plant yourself under any circumstances, as European centaury, like all other members of the gentian family, is on the list of protected plants!

Cultivation

Raising European centaury in your herb garden is not recommended.

European Cowslip: The Remedy of Choice for Old Age Cough

Whenever a stubborn cough needs treatment, a case in which the coughing up of viscid secretions is proving difficult, medicinal plants with a high saponin content are particularly helpful.

Taken in the form of a tea, they liquefy the viscid bronchial mucus, which thus becomes easier to bring up by coughing. The roots of the European cowslip are rich in saponins of this kind; they contain 5 to 10 percent triterpene saponins. For this reason, European cowslip roots are a major ingredient of any tea used as a cough remedy. They are especially successful with chronic coughs in older people, the so-called old age cough. These coughs are often caused by decreased cardiac efficiency, which leads to pulmonary congestion and thus to a tickle in the throat and phlegm production. To be of help here, it is necessary not only to loosen the phlegm for easier expectoration, but also to lessen the strain on the circulatory system by promoting increased elimination of water. That is precisely the effect of European cowslip roots in a tea for coughs; they loosen phlegm and remove water.

The German Office of Health lists catarrhs of the respiratory passages as the area of application for the European cowslip.

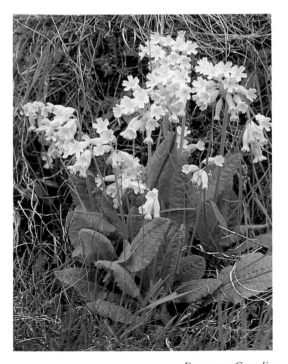

European Cowslip

Botanically the true European cowslip is known as *Primula veris* L., also as *Primula officinalis*. Its common names include fairycup, keyflower, key of heaven, and paigle. It grows principally in meadows, where it is anchored in the ground with a rhizome that produces a great many fibrous roots. The basal leaves are oblong to ovate, and their undersides are hairy. The leaf blade narrows toward the base. The flowers grow in umbels at the ends of stalks of varying lengths. The calyx is whitish-green and squared; the corolla is tubular, flared at the top, and yellow, with a deep golden-yellow tone in the center. Often European cowslips bloom as early as March, though April is more usual.

Two different species, *Primula elatior*, the woodland cowslip, and *Primula vulgaris*, are primroses also used for pharmaceutical purposes. They are no less efficacious than the true European cowslip.

Cultivation
Raising the medicinally useful European cowslip in your own garden is not recommended. In ornamental gardens, however, the cultivated varieties of the various primrose species are highly decorative in springtime.

Eyebright: Strengthens Sickly Children

This plant was unknown in classical antiquity because it did not grow in Greece, but it is mentioned in the first German book on medicinal herbs published in 1485.

Science has paid scant attention to eyebright; its use is confined to folk medicine, whose practitioners swear by its beneficial effect on eye inflammations and coughs and its ability to give strength to sickly children. It appears that the body's powers of resistance are activated by eyebright tea.

Various *Euphrasia* species—primarily *Euphrasia officinalis* and *Euphrasia rostkoviana* with all their subspecies and hybrids—provide us with eyebright tea. *Euphrasia*, which belongs to the botanical family of the Scrophulariaceae,

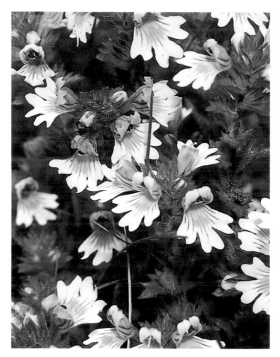

Eyebright

or snapdragons, grows semiparasitically in meadows, on sunny slopes, in heathland, and in open woods in mountainous regions. The plant can reach a height of 4 to 8 inches (10–20 cm) or up to 12 inches (30 cm). Its upper portion has profusely branching stems, is covered with downy hairs, and bears sharply serrate leaves in opposite pairs. In the leaf axils, especially those of the upper leaves, grow pale violet (also white) flowers with a lower three-lobed lip. Eyebright blooms in late summer or in fall.

It is harvested during the blooming season, made into bundles for drying, and hung in a well-ventilated place. Used internally in a course of treatment with tea and externally as a wash, eyebright is said to be an effective acne remedy.

Cultivation
Eyebright, a semiparasite, is quite difficult to raise and tend in your own garden. Cultivating it is therefore not recommended.

Fennel: One of Our Oldest Medicinal Plants and Culinary Herbs

We are fairly certain that fennel was in use over 4000 years ago. It is even mentioned in the famous Ebers Papyrus, an ancient Egyptian collection of medical writings made around 1500 B.C. There it is referred to principally as a remedy for flatulence. Later authors of herbals, such as Pliny (A.D. 23–79), also describe fennel primarily as an aid to digestion.

In the Middle Ages, however, fennel seeds were also praised as a superb remedy for coughs and stubborn mucus. These therapeutic indications, along with the efficacy of fennel in treating gastric and intestinal problems, are of great significance even today. The German Office of Health, in recommending the application of fennel, refers expressly to its ability to dissolve mucus in the respiratory passages.

Fennel is native to the Mediterranean area, where it can be found growing wild. To meet the huge demand for high-quality fennel seeds, fennel has long been cultivated—for use in medicinal preparations, as a vegetable, or as a culinary herb—in the warmer parts of Europe and in many parts of Africa, Asia, and North and South America.

Fennel is an annual or perennial; it grows 39 to 79 inches (1–2 m) tall and is anchored in the soil by a fleshy root. Its terete stem is finely ridged, covered with a blue bloom, and profusely branched at the top. The tips of the feathery, much-divided leaves are quite narrow; the middle and upper leaves have large sheaths. The tiny yellow fennel flowers are arranged in double umbels. The umbel and the umbellet have no small involucral leaves. Fennel blooms from July until September. It is striking that the fruits (seeds) do not ripen at the same time, either within the same cultivated area or on a single plant. This makes the harvesting of the seeds in fields quite expensive. First, workers go through the fields to cut out the ripened umbels. This process is called "combing." Because it is done with great care, the comb fennel is of extremely high quality. Later, the plants are torn from the ground in their entirety and threshed. The seeds—actually dehiscent fruits—fall apart into two mesocarps when dried. Fennel is sold in this form, and it should be stored in this form as well. The fruits (seeds) contain about 7 percent essential oil consisting largely of an ethole (60 percent) and d-fenchone (20 percent). It is advisable to crush the seeds in a mortar before preparing the tea, because this releases more essential oil from them.

Fennel, known to botanists as *Foeniculum vulgare*, belongs to the carrot family (Apiaceae-Umbelliferae). The fleshy root and lower stem and stalk portions of one cultivated variety are eaten as a vegetable.

Salad lovers are advised to try fennel weed, the fresh leaf tips of the fennel plant; they have a refreshing taste. With a mixture of dill weed and fennel weed you can season cucumber salad and a variety of lettuce salads, as well as vegetable soups and stews. Fennel seeds make fresh bread more nourishing.

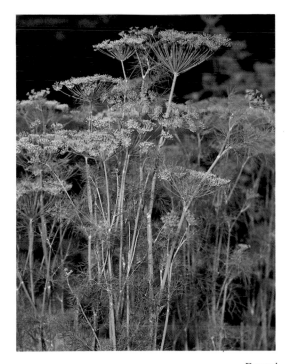

Fennel

Cultivation

If you enjoy harvesting your own fennel seeds, then I can only encourage you to do so. You will need plenty of room in your herb garden, however, as fennel plants grow quite tall. In mid-April put the seed into humus soil. Sow the seeds in rows spaced about 8 inches (20 cm) apart, so that the plants have room to develop. Choose a sunny location. If you water them diligently, the seeds will sprout after two or three weeks. Then the young fennel has to be thinned out so that the plants are 3 to 4 inches (8–10 cm) apart.

Once winter is approaching, cut off the plants at hand's height above the ground and cover them with peat and pine brush to prevent freezing. In the second year, you can harvest the seeds. If you remember to water, you will have an abundant harvest. To keep the plants from falling over (when the wind blows), stake them well in advance. Fennel seeds do not ripen at the same time; for this reason, from August on keep cutting off the shoots that contain ripe seeds. You can tell the ripe shoots by their brown color. Dry the umbels in the open air in a little gauze bag, until the seeds fall off when you shake the bag (see Proper Harvesting and Careful Preparation, page 138).

Flax: Known from Time Immemorial

Linum usitatissimum is the botanical name of this plant in the flax fmaily (Linaceae), which is commonly known also as linseed or lint bells. As early as the Mesolithic period, it was known to man for its usefulness. In that era, flax provided both oil and fiber for garments, as the remains of prehistoric lake dwellers in Switzerland indicate. The cultivation of flax in Egypt can be traced back to the fourteenth century B.C.; flaxseed intended as provisions for the last journey was found in Egyptian burial chambers. In the writings of Hippocrates (around 500 B.C.) flaxseed is first mentioned as a remedy for catarrhs, stomachache, and diarrhea. And Theophrastus von Hohenheim—called Paracelsus (1493–1541)—refers to flaxseed mucilage as a soothing cough remedy.

The use of flaxseed in folk medicine probably started in Germany. Hieronymus Bock reported at great length on the medicinal use of flaxseed in his herbal of the year 1577: "Flaxseed crushed and pulverized, mixed with some pepper and honey to form an electuary, soothes a cough and brings pleasure to the works of Nature. Should any man's insides be inflamed, you may boil flaxseed in water for him, mix honey with it and give it to him to drink. . . . Flaxseed softens, soothes, and stops all fiery swellings, inside and outside. . . ."

Today flaxseed is used for self medication as a regulative to treat sluggishness of the bowels and constipation. The German Office of Health

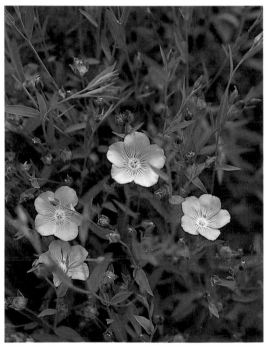

Flax

lists the following areas of application for flaxseed: Bulk-forming laxative to relieve constipation and functional intestinal disorders; in the form of mucilage preparations as an adjunct to the treatment of inflammatory gastric and intestinal disorders. Ground flaxseed (flaxseed meal) has long been used to make hot poultices for external application where heat is needed.

The flaxseed used for medicinal purposes contains mucilage, pectin, fatty oil with polyunsaturated fatty acids and linamarin, a hydrocyanic acid glycoside. The fear that the hydrocyanic acid content could cause poisoning, particularly if used over a long period, is unfounded. This side effect has never been observed, because when flaxseed is eaten, the enzyme linase—which releases the hydrocyanic acid—is rendered inactive in the acid environment of the stomach.

With the assistance of the cellulose contained in the seed coat, mucilage—which accounts for 3 to 6 percent of the contents of the seed coat—stimulates peristaltic motion, particularly in the colon, and this leads to evacuation. Fat and mucilage act as lubricants. The mucilage content is also responsible for the effectiveness of flaxseed in treating inflammatory gastric and intestinal disorders.

Flax, which grows 12 to 31 inches (30–80 cm) high, is known only as a cultivated plant. The stem usually is erect and branches only at the inflorescence. The alternate leaves, which may be as long as 1.6 inches (4 cm), are narrow and pointed. The light-blue flowers, with their five sepals, grow singly at the ends of the lateral branches. From these flowers the fruit (seedpod) ripens into a rounded capsule with five compartments. The seeds are ovate, flat, shiny, brown, and 5 to 6 millimeters long.

Cultivation

Flax can be grown in your garden as an ornamental (from seed sown in spring). The seeds can be obtained only with field cultivation.

Fumitory: Once in Frequent Use, Now Rediscovered

Fumaria officinalis L., also known as earthsmoke, a member of the Papaveraceae or poppy family, is a delicate, pretty plant. Its flowers and leaves are particularly attractive. Fumitory generally grows erect to a height of 8 to 16 inches (20–40 cm), but in some places it is decumbent. The hollow stems are smooth, have a bluish bloom, and branch profusely. Alternate, gray-green leaves grow on the upper part of the plant. The lower leaves are stalked and bipinnate to tripinnate, with tiny, narrow pinnules. The spurred flowers, arranged in loose clusters (racemes), are pink to dark red. This medicinal plant, which prefers landfills, fallow land, gardens, and farmland, blooms in June and July.

Fumitory was mentioned by the Roman writer Pliny (A.D. 23–79) and by Dioscorides (a Greek physician of the first century A.D.). In the first herbal published in German, it was praised as a diuretic, a gallbladder remedy, and a cure for

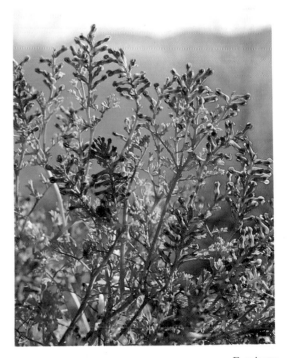

Fumitory

constipation. For a long time thereafter fumitory was forgotten or seldom used, but then scientists rediscovered it as a substance that acts "against cramplike pain in the area of the gallbladder and the bile ducts as well as the gastrointestinal tract" (German Office of Health). Today the drug is a common ingredient of depurative teas and gallbladder, liver, and stomach teas. The tea applications used to treat skin eruptions are also being revived. Significantly, one of fumitory's common German names once was scabweed. The aerial parts of the plant are used for medicinal purposes.

Cultivation

Gardens are among the natural habitats of fumitory. If fumitory "sneaks" into your orchard, herb garden, or vegetable garden, grant it asylum there—partly to enjoy its flowers and leaves, partly to become familiar with and try out its curative effect.

Gentian: Its Bitter Chemical Substances Make It Popular

"Medicine has to taste bitter; otherwise, it's no good!" This remark, in earlier times often applied to medicinal plants that keep the digestive tract in good working order, is still valid for gentian today. Bitter constituents, aromatic bitter constituents, or acrid constituents cause the glands that produce peptic juice to increase their output, which in turn stimulates the appetite and accelerates the assimilation of nutrients, so that gas pains and feelings of pressure and fullness after meals never even get underway. In particular, digestive insufficiency (the sluggish process of digestion due to old age) in older people is noticeably improved by this "bitter medicine." Gentian is one of the pure bitter agents, the *Amara tonica,* and has a high content of bitter chemical substances. The German Office of Health recommends tea made from gentian roots as a remedy for digestive problems such as lack of appetite, a feeling of fullness, and flatulence. It is contraindicated, however, where gastric and intestinal ulcers are present. The species used for medicinal purposes, known as *Gentiana lutea,* is a yellow (as "lutea" indicates) gentian. I want to emphasize here that several gentian species are on the list of protected plants and may not be collected.

Gentiana lutea, once considered a pesky weed by mountain farmers, is a stately herbaceous plant that grows about 39 inches (1 m) tall. The bare, erect stem is hollow and bears large decussate, elliptical, bluish-green leaves crisscrossed with prominent arched veins. The leaf stalks become progressively shorter toward the top of the plant. Yellow gentian is anchored in the ground with a long, strong root. It takes several years for the plant to yield its yellow flowers, which are arranged in dense false whorls. The blooming period is July to September.

The beauty of this plant was not the sole cause of its becoming a rarity. It was dug up with increasing frequency for use in making enzian, a spirit distilled from its roots. Not only the yellow gentian was decimated, but also other, blue-flowering, species with sufficiently large roots.

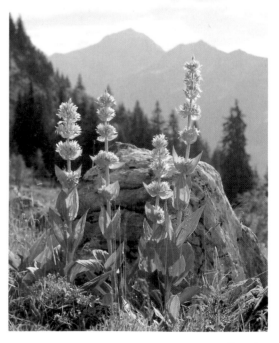

Genetian

Cultivation

Through a garden center you can purchase a yellow gentian as an ornamental for your garden, but raising this plant for its roots is not recommended.

Goldenrod: Famed as a Bladder and Kidney Remedy Since the Middle Ages

When the summer's showy display of flowers is coming to a close, goldenrod is beginning to bloom along the edges of forests, on embankments, in dry meadows, in forest clearings, on cutover land, and along roadsides, wherever the sun finds unimpeded access. Its tiny flower heads, which grow in simple clusters or in panicled clusters, are bright yellow. They smell faintly aromatic.

Botanists call this medicinal plant *Solidago virgaurea* and classify it as a member of the composite family (Asteraceae = Compositae). Medicinal use is made of all the parts above the ground, although in harvesting you should give preference to the flowering region and leave the lignified lower parts of this plant, which grows over 20 inches (50 cm) tall.

There is little that tells us with certainty whether goldenrod was already in use in antiquity. One clue passed on to us by Hieronymus Bock (1592), refers to the Teutons; they used goldenrod as a vulnerary herb.

Since the Middle Ages, goldenrod has been esteemed as a bladder and kidney medicine, and today this medicinal plant still is held to be effective in treating inflammations of the bladder, kidneys, and urinary passages. If your doctor advises you to drink plenty of liquids, these can include goldenrod tea. Teas used in courses of treatment in spring and fall also contain the aerial parts of goldenrod.

The German Office of Health recommends goldenrod to increase urine flow in treating bladder and kidney inflammations. On the basis of its stimulating effect on overall body metabolism, goldenrod also has been tried in cases of rheumatism and gout. The reports on these

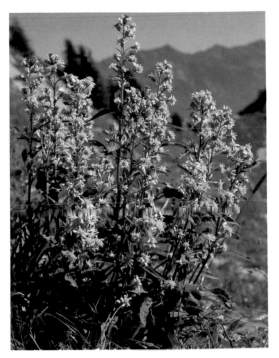

Goldenrod

experiments are encouraging, but scientists as yet know of no active substances that justify application for these purposes.

In addition to the goldenrod described here—true goldenrod, as I would like to call it to distinguish it from the others—two other *Solidago* species grow wild and in our gardens as well: *Solidago canadensis* and *Solidago gigantea ssp. serotina*. Their active substances closely resemble those of true goldenrod. *Solidago canadensis* is commonly used as a medicinal plant in North America. *Solidago virgaurea,* which is of acknowledged medicinal benefit, has not yet been recommended for pharmaceutical use.

Cultivation

Nothing is easier than growing goldenrod in your garden. From a garden store or from friends, get some cuttings and set them in a sunny location in spring or late fall. Make sure the site you choose does not permit standing water to collect, even after a prolonged rainfall. Goldenrod does not like wet roots. Otherwise, it will thrive in normal garden soil and needs very little care: If you occasionally turn up and loosen the soil around the plant, this will be enough.

When buying these herbaceous plants in the garden store, make sure you get true goldenrod, which bears the botanical name *Solidago virgaurea*.

Harvest the upper flowering tops in summer at the start of the blooming season, dry them in the open air, and cut them into small pieces. Then store them where light and dampness cannot reach them (see page 12).

Giant goldenrod (*Solidago gigantea ssp. serotina*) and Canadian goldenrod (*Solidago canadense*) also have become naturalized in this country as ornamentals.

Goutweed: A Garden Weed

Scarcely any modern-day books of medicinal plants still list goutweed (*Aegopodium podagraria*), also known as goutwort, ashweed,

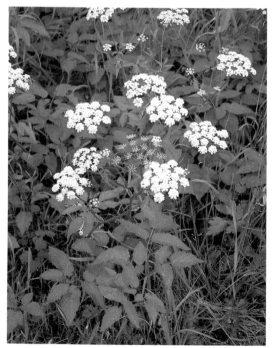

Goutweed

ground elder, bishop's weed, and herb Gerarde, as a medicinal herb. Nevertheless, its Latin name and its English common name contain references to the fact that this garden weed, which riots in great abundance along fences, was once a valued remedy for gout: Podagra is an older term for gout in the big toe.

Goutweed, a member of the carrot family (Apiaceae = Umbelliferae), is a herbaceous plant with long stolons that proliferate under the ground. On the erect stalks, 12 to 31.5 inches (30–80 cm) tall, grow simply to doubly pinnate leaves, which, with their large, sometimes doubly serrate leaf segments, resemble a goat's foot. The double umbels have 15 to 25 ligules, without involucral leaves and small phyllaries. The blooming season extends from May into November.

Folk medicine used—and now once again uses—the fresh leaves, which are crushed and placed on the aching, swollen gouty concretions to ease the pain. Gout sufferers also are said to be helped by eating a vegetable dish made from the fresh leaves of goutweed, prepared like spinach; in addition, the dried leaves are used as a tea to treat rheumatism (*Preparation*, see page 75).

Cultivation
If your garden is not "sterile," you need not worry about raising goutweed. It grows everywhere: along fences, between the beds, and even in orchards. Growing it directly in herb beds is really not necessary.

> **Please note**
> Goutweed belongs to the carrot family, which also includes poisonous species. Please use this plant only if you can identify it with certainty!

Hawthorn: Strengthens Heart and Nerves

The hawthorn genus (*Crataegus*), which belongs to the rose family (Rosaceae), includes shrubs or small trees that have sharp thorns on their

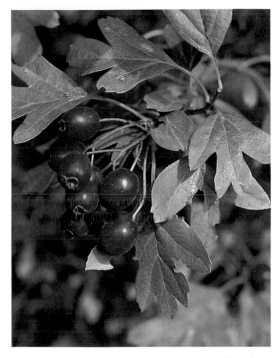

Hawthorn

Hawthorn has played a role as a medicinal plant only since the turn of the century. Its effect has been studied thoroughly by scientists, and the area of application has been clearly outlined: It aids older and aged people who have the "overstrained heart of old age," and it helps "stressed" people who have overtaxed hearts, diminished efficiency, and feelings of pressure and constriction in the cardiac region, as well as people with milder forms of cardiac arrhythmia.

A tea made from hawthorn flowers or from a mixture of hawthorn flowers and leaves is—if applied in a course of treatment—an invigorating source of comfort for the overburdened heart. It has been proved that no side effects need be feared, even if the tea is drunk over an extended period.

A course of treatment with tea also is recommended after recovery from a heart attack. Moreover, the theory that hawthorn may possibly prevent myocardial infarctions cannot be brushed aside.

The hypotensive effect attributed to hawthorn, however, is controversial. It can be used only as an adjunct therapy in efforts to lower blood pressure.

The active substances of hawthorn have been studied, but the action cannot be ascribed to any one of its constituents alone. The primary effect doubtless is due to procyanidins, flavonoids, amines, and phenolic acids.

The German Office of Health lists the following areas of application for hawthorn tea: Diminished efficiency of an aging heart that is not yet in need of digitalis; feelings of pressure and constriction in the cardiac region; mild forms of cardiac arrhythmia.

Cultivation

Hawthorn shrubs, which you can buy at a nursery, flourish best in loose, permeable, slightly loamy soils. They like sun, but if necessary can also tolerate shady locations. Once your hawthorn shrub has taken hold in your garden, you need not worry further, as this plant is not sensitive and lives to a ripe old age. If it grows too tall, you can cut it back to keep it shrubby.

branches. The white flowers, which occur in erect umbellike panicles, bloom in May or June in indescribable abundance. The flowers and thorns gave the plant one of its English common names, whitethorn. Other names are English hawthorn, haw, and maybush.

Hawthorn grows in thin underbrush and hedges; it is also frequently found on sunny slopes and in open woods.

For pharmaceutical purposes, the parts used are the flowers, leaves, and fruits of various *Crataegus* species, of which the most important are *Crataegus laevigata*, the English hawthorn, and *Crataegus monogyna*, the one-seed hawthorn.

Although medieval herbals often tell us otherwise, we have to assume that hawthorn was not in use in ancient times, at least not as a tonic for the weakened hearts of older people. It seems certain only that the *Sirupus Senelorum* of the personal physician of Henry IV of France (1553–1610) was a syrup made from hawthorn fruits.

(Hawthorn shrubs are a shelterwood and feeding place for birds!)

In spring, hawthorn develops a luxuriant array of white flowers, and in fall, bright-red fruits appear, slightly reminiscent of rose hips, the fruits of the dog rose. Even a layman can tell by the fruits that the hawthorn belongs to the rose family. The flowers and the young leaves yield an excellent tea. The flowers are harvested right after they open; the leaves, when they are completely developed. Quickly dry what you have collected and store it in containers that can be tightly closed.

Hayseed: Often Used by Pastor Kneipp

Hayseed is a mixture of flower parts, seeds, and smallish pieces of leaves and stems of various grasses and meadow flowers that were dried along with the hay. In earlier times, it was simply picked up off the threshing floor—it included everything that the pitchfork couldn't get

and that settled in an increasingly thick layer on the barn floor. Before being used for pharmaceutical purposes, the hayseed was sifted to remove coarse stem parts and soil.

Along with typical meadow grasses like couch grass, brome, meadow cockle, and meadow fescue, hayseed also contains parts of other meadow plants. Different batches of hayseed vary widely in their composition, depending on the amounts of the meadow plants they contain. That probably was why the curative effect of hayseed was not scientifically recognized for a great many years. Pastor Kneipp (the Swiss "Water Doctor": 1821–1897), however, already was convinced of its medicinal value and used it often.

Hayseed poultices and baths alleviate pain, calm and relax cramped muscles, improve the elasticity of connective tissue, step up circulation, and increase tissue metabolism.

Hayseed baths and even the old hayseed applications such as hayseed packs and hayseed shirts help to heighten the body's powers of resistance and are used successfully to treat

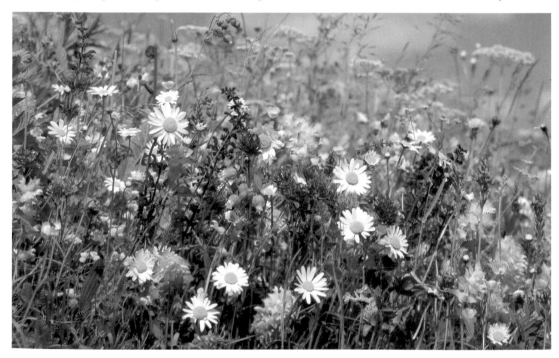

Hayseed

flulike infections (colds) accompanied by fever. Hayseed baths have been quite helpful with rheumatism also. They are praised for their alterative effect in treating states of restlessness during menopause and for their effect on various symptoms of neurodystonia. Even chronic skin problems and stomach, intestinal, bladder, and kidney ailments respond well to hayseed poultices and to full and partial hayseed baths.

Thus far no special active substances have been found in hayseed that would account for its soothing effect. It contains substances that usually are present in varying amounts in all plants: sugar, minerals and trace elements, proteins, starch, tannins, and a little essential oil. In addition, hayseed contains flavonoids and coumarin—possibly it owes its healing effect to these substances.

Cultivation

Raising hayseed yourself is not applicable in this case.

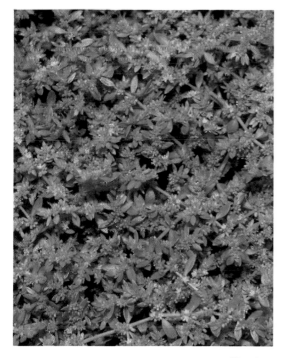

Herniary

Herniary: Popular Only in Folk Medicine

Experience teaches us that a kidney and bladder tea is more effective if it contains herniary, along with other herbs that disinfect the kidneys, bladder, and urinary passages and bring about an increase in urination: Cramplike pain is alleviated. That is the reason herniary is still in use.

The rationale for the negative attitude of the German Office of Health is as follows: Because there is insufficient evidence of its efficacy in the areas of application in question, therapeutic application cannot be recommended.

Indeed, there are a great many applications in folk medicine in which herniary certainly is not particularly helpful: illnesses that affect the respiratory passages (coughs and asthma), neuritis, rheumatism and gout, jaundice, and gallbladder problems. It does, however, have an antispasmodic effect on the urinary passages, and it is useful in depurative teas as a metabolic stimulant—provided that no contraindications are known to be present. Saponins are known to be present in herniary.

Herniary, which has the botanical name *Herniaria glabra* (smooth herniary) or *Herniaria hirsuta* (hairy herniary), is also known as rupture wort, a member of the pink family (Caryophyllaceae). This information will surely come as a surprise to you, as the plants bear no visible similarity to the pinks or carnations we know so well. These inconspicuous decumbent herbs seem almost to cling to the ground, and their flowers are small and unassuming.

Both species of herniary are among the most common plants of our native flora, but because of their unobtrusiveness few people know their name, and even herb lovers overlook them. Herniary grows chiefly along paths and in sandy fields, pastures, landfills, and rocky wasteland.

The stem of smooth herniary is hairless, that of hairy herniary, covered with hair. On both types of stems grow small elliptical or lanceolate opposite leaflets 3 to 8 millimeters long. The tiny little flowers (rarely larger than 1 millimeter) grow in a convoluted arrangement of five to

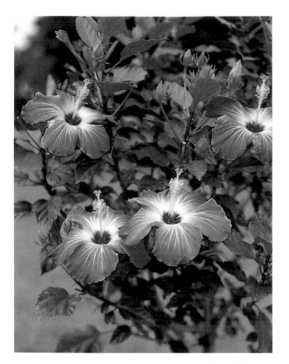

Hibiscus Flowers

Hibiscus flowers have a refreshingly tart taste, produced by organic acids, citric acid, hibiscic acid, malic acid, tartaric acid, large amounts of ascorbic acid (= vitamin C), and pigments, which chiefly determine the use of this tea drug and give the blossoms their color. Whenever a tea needs a refreshing note, a more attractive appearance, or a tart taste, we reach for the hibiscus flowers.

In recent times, scientists have paid rather more attention to the substances contained in this popular tea drug. The tea is conceded to be slightly diuretic; mention is made of an antispasmodic property; and there is talk of an ability to combat intestinal worms. A slight antibacterial effect has also been found to exist. All this is not sufficient, however, to grant hibiscus flowers the status of a healing drug, such as chamomile, for example. The flowers, however, do markedly improve the taste of all tea blends to which they are added.

Cultivation

Hibiscus can be grown in southern California and Florida. Raising hibiscus yourself in colder regions is possible only as container plants. Outdoors, choose a sunny location that is sheltered from wind. Water abundantly, but avoid standing water. Overwinter in a bright place about 57 to 61°F (14–16°C) and water little. Cut back any stems that have become too long in the spring of the second year.

ten blossoms close together. The tiny greenish-yellow flowers bloom from June to September.

Cultivation

If you find several specimens of this "weed"—as garden owners generally call it—growing in your garden, grant them asylum. I cannot advise you to raise herniary, however, because it is not particularly suitable for household use.

Hibiscus Flowers: A Refreshing Taste

In herb and spice shops they are sold under the name of Nubia flowers, red mallow, African mallow, carcade, or roselle—all these terms refer to hibiscus flowers. These are the dried calyxes and outer calyxes—harvested during fruiting season—of *Hibiscus sabdariffa* L., a shrubby member of the mallow family (Malvaceae) that is probably native to Africa but grows also in China, Mexico, Thailand, and the Sudan.

High Mallow: A Medicinal Plant Rich in Soothing Mucilage

According to a medieval herbal, Pliny said that "whosoever shall take a drink of the juice of cheeses (meaning high mallows, also commonly known as cheeseflowers or fairy cheeses) shall that day be free from all diseases that shall come to him." A great compliment for a medicinal plant—but even high mallow is no miracle drug, no universal remedy. In folk medicine it soon became clear what the primary areas of application are: catarrhs of the upper respiratory

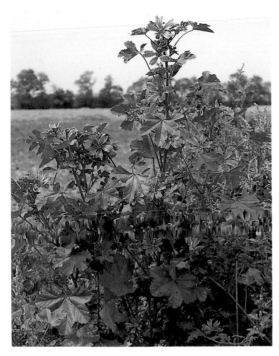

High Mallow

always bear long-stalked, usually five-lobed leaves, which are downy on both sides and crenate, or scalloped, along the edges. In the leaf axils grow long, hairy pedicels that bear bluish to rose-pink flowers at their ends. The five petals are deeply crenate and display three dark longitudinal stripes. The blooming period is June, July, and August. That is also the time for harvesting. Gather the flowers with the calyx but without the stalk; the leaves; or even all the parts above the ground.

Please note

Hibiscus sabdariffa L., which supplies us with hibiscus flowers (see page 176), is also a member of the Malvaceae or mallow family, but not comparable with our high mallow. The hibiscus is valued for its refreshing fruit acids and its vitamin C; the high mallow, also known as the blue mallow, or common mallow, is esteemed for the soothing mucins.

Cultivation

This member of the mallow family is suitable for raising in your backyard garden, but can become invasive.

passages, including coughs, hoarseness, and sore throat, and catarrhs in the gastrointestinal region. High mallow leaves contain about 8 percent plant mucilage, high mallow flowers, about 10 percent. This substance soothes by forming a protective coating over inflamed mucous membranes. The tannin content as well as flavonoids adds to the effect. In the package circular for high mallow tea (stipulated by the German Office of Health) the following areas of application are listed: Inflammation of the mucous membranes in the mouth and throat area as well as in the gastrointestinal region; catarrhs of the upper respiratory passages.

Malva silvestris L., family Malvaceae, is the botanical name of the mallow species used for pharmaceutical purposes. It grows along roadsides, in landfills, along field and meadow paths, and on slopes and walls. There are a great many other mallow species, but they play a role only in folk medicine. *Malva silvestris* is anchored in the ground with a spindle-shaped root. From it arise several branchy, hairy stems, which may be erect, ascending, or even decumbent. They

Hop: Known as a Beer Additive

Hop is known as one of the most important ingredients of beer and as a medicinal herb: a tranquilizer, a soporific, and a remedy for stomach upsets. Indeed, these are the major areas of application for this plant, known to botanists as *Humulus lupulus*, a member of the hemp family (Cannabinaceae). It reputedly originated in eastern Europe, but since the eighth century it has been common throughout central Europe.

Hop is a perennial vine reaching up to approximately 10 to 20 feet (3–6 m) in length. The stalk of this right-hand twiner has climbing hairs and is covered with long-stemmed, three- to five-lobed, extremely coarse opposite leaves. Male and female blossoms are located on different plants of this dioecious vine. Medicinally and for purposes of brewing beer, only the

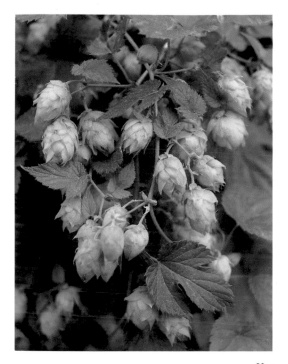

Hop

Today hops are used in three ways: as aromatic bitters to treat lack of appetite, weak stomachs, and nervous gastric disorders; as a tranquilizer for people in an overwrought state or suffering from sleep disturbances, nervous agitation, and sexual hyperexcitability; and in folk medicine, externally, as a compress for ulcers and suppurating wounds.

The substances contained in hop have been, for the most part, thoroughly investigated. Three groups determine the medicinal effect: The essential oil, which makes up 0.3 to 1.0 percent of the hop cones, has been subjected to particularly extensive research as the vehicle for the aromatic substances. More than 150 individual components have been discovered in it. The essential oil plays no obvious role in the sedative effect of the hop cones, but it might contribute to the antibacterial effect attributed to hop. Tannins, which constitute 2 to 4 percent of the hop cones, justify the application of hop to combat diarrhea and intestinal disorders accompanied by foul-smelling diarrhea and intestinal gas. The bitters humulon and lupulon make hop cones an effective stomachic. They also account for the sedative effect, and they exhibit antibiotic activity. During storage, oxidation causes a substance (2-methyl-3-butene diol) to split off from the bitter constituents; a sedative effect is attributed to it. We assume that when hop tea is prepared and drunk, conversion of humulon and lupulon takes place; this might explain the sedative effect. Surely, though, additional substances contained in hop play some role in its action. The sedative action of hop baths and herbal pillows may be considered a certainty.

The German Office of Health recommends tea made from hop cones for conditions of ill health such as restlessness and sleep disturbances.

Cultivation
Although it is possible to grow hops in your backyard, I advise against it because it is too involved.

flowers of the female plants are used, the hop cones, which are cultivated on a large scale. The hop shoots climb up ascending wires and produce inflorescences thickly covered with flowers, with the individual flowers arranged in false spikes. From these inflorescences develop the hop cones.

The medicinal use of hop cones has a very long history. It is interesting, however, that in the Middle Ages they were used not as a sedative, but as a remedy for gallbladder and liver complaints, a stomachic, a diuretic, and a laxative.

We know that the Romans valued young hop shoots as a wholesome vegetable, and that use has continued to the present time. Today "hop asparagus" is prepared as a vegetable dish or minced and added to salads. As an ingredient of pancake batter, fresh hop shoots are considered a delicacy. Pietro A. Mathioli (1501–1577) writes of hop asparagus: "In spring gourmets have the young hop asparagus prepared as a salad—and think it a good food for clogged livers."

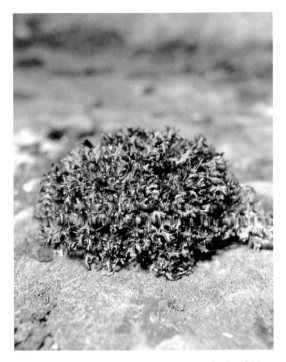

Iceland Moss

Today Iceland moss is in demand again as a tea drug also, primarily for irritations in the throat area and for the dry cough that often appears at the start of a flulike infection. Iceland moss, however, is also effective against gastritis, lack of appetite, and debility following recovery from infectious diseases, because along with large amounts of plant mucilage, bitter lichenic acids—shown to possess an antibiotic effect—also have been found in the drug.

The German Office of Health, more reserved in its recommendations, endorses the use of Iceland moss solely to soothe irritated mucous membranes in catarrhs affecting the upper respiratory passages.

Botanists call Iceland moss *Cetraria islandica.* It grows as a shrub in humus and sandy soils, especially in mountainous areas, to a height of 1.5 to almost 5 inches (4–12 cm). The lichen grows squarrose, forked, or branched like antlers. The leaflike individual shoots are 5 to 20 millimeters across, but usually curled or grooved and crooked. The upper surface (turned toward the light) is olive to brownish green, the lower surface (turned away from the light) is whitish green to light brownish, often with white spots.

Iceland Moss: An Old Medicinal Plant Rediscovered

To set things right at the very outset: The English common name "Iceland moss" is botanically incorrect. This plant is not a moss at all, but a lichen, a symbiosis (mutually beneficial relationship) made up of a fungus and an alga. The name has been employed as long as the plant has been in medicinal use—that is, since the seventeenth century. Since that time, Iceland moss has been one of the best-loved medicinal plants in the realm of folk medicine, especially as a treatment for pulmonary and bronchial trouble. This history is reflected in other common names: lung moss, cough moss, and fever moss. In our century this medicinal plant, like many others, fell into obscurity. Only the gelatinous Iceland moss tablets were able to hold their own as a remedy for sore throat and hoarseness.

Cultivation
This medicinal plant is virtually impossible to raise in your own garden.

Juniper Berries: Effective Against Rheumatism, But Not Without Side Effects

It was Sebastian Kneipp who recommended juniper berries as a remedy for rheumatism and gout, and since that time the juniper berry treatment has been applied in folk medicine.

Common juniper is known by botanists as *Juniperus communis* L. It belongs to the cypress family (Cupressaceae). Its accessory fruits (pseudocarps), small berrylike cones, provide us with the flavoring and pharmaceutical drug.

Juniper, a decumbent shrub or a columnar tree with accumbent branches, grows on mountain

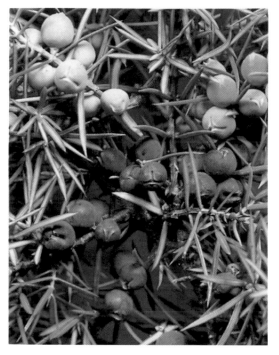

Juniper Berries

about 1 to 2 percent, the composition of which is quite complex. The oil also is the source of the side effects, as certain substances in this essential oil—namely alpha-pinene and beta-pinene—can severely irritate the kidneys.

> **Please note**
> Although this danger can virtually be ruled out when the juniper berries are eaten or used as a flavoring, it is nonetheless inadvisable to use the berries if kidney damage is present or during pregnancy.

The German Office of Health is reserved in its assessment of the range of effectiveness of juniper berries. Despite positive experiences with application to treat chronic rheumatism and to increase urine flow, juniper berries are recommended for use only in treating digestive disturbances such as belching, heartburn, and a feeling of fullness.

Cultivation
Juniper is a common ornamental shrub that is easily grown and can be obtained from any nursery.

slopes, heaths, and moors, and as underbrush in clear woods and pastures. Its stiff, pointed leaves, the needles, are about .4 inch (1 cm) long. They occur in threes or, less often, in fours and appear together in whorls. The flowers are dioecious; female and male flowers appear only on different plants. Because they are green and plain, they attract little attention. After fertilization, the berrylike fruits begin to ripen; it takes three years for them to mature fully. Ripe fruits are spherical, blue-black, and 5 to 8 millimeters in diameter. The triradiate cleft is a reminder that the "juniper berries"—according to their botanical description—are really cones. Because of the sharp leaf prickles (leaves formed in the shape of needles), it is virtually impossible to pick the berries. Therefore people resort to other means: They spread out cloths on the ground, knock the ripe berries off, and pick them up off the cloth. The trade designation "Italian" means that the berries are large and fully ripened, not necessarily that they are of Italian origin.

The most important active substance in juniper berries is without doubt the essential oil,

Lavender: Popular for Its Fragrance

At one time lavender grew in every ornamental garden: Our great-great-grandmothers held this "most delightfully" scented medicinal plant in great esteem. They hung sachets of lavender flowers in the clothes closets and, on festive occasions, tucked one into their corsets too. A lavender bath was one of the most favored perfumed baths. Then, for a time, lavender was not much talked about. Today, however, it has regained its great popularity.

Lavender is native to the western Mediterranean area, but it quickly reached the regions north of the Alps, where it thrives splendidly in ornamental gardens and herb gardens.

This plant's botanical names are *Lavandula officinalis, Lavandula angustifolia,* and *Lavandula spica.* It belongs to the mint family

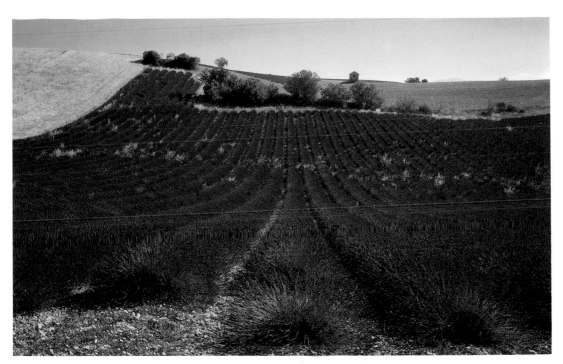

Lavender

(Lamiaceae = Labiatae), to which many other, for the most part sweet-smelling, medicinal plants belong, including lemon balm, peppermint, sage, and thyme.

The lavender used for medicinal purposes generally is cultivated, and this ensures that no flowers other than those of *Lavandula officinalis* are employed, as there are a great many strains and subspecies.

Lavender grows up to 24 inches (60 cm) tall. The erect branches of this subshrub bear opposite, linear to lanceolate, entire gray-green leaves that are involuted along the margins. The lower leaves are covered on both sides with white felt-like hairs. The violet flowers are borne on peduncles in false whorls, which form an interrupted spike. Each false whorl consists of six to ten flowers. The blooming season is July to August.

The altogether pleasant-smelling essential oil of the flowers is lavender's primary active agent. Others are coumarins, triterpenes, and flavonoids. Lavender flowers act on the central nervous system as a sedative and also soothe the bronchial tubes. In the stomach and intestines they relieve cramps, disinfect, and stimulate the flow of gastric juice. Usually lavender is an ingredient of tea blends prescribed for various states of nervous tension. Lavender baths are good for people with hypotonicity (overly low blood pressure) because it refreshes them, and for people who are irritable and under stress because it relaxes them. Spirit of lavender (from the pharmacy) was once frequently used to allay the pain of rheumatism.

Lavender is valued not only as a medicinal plant, but also as a pleasant seasoning in combination with dill, basil, thyme, or summer savory. Please use it sparingly to season, so that the scent is just barely perceptible, never dominant.

The German Office of Health attests that the tea made from lavender flowers helps conditions such as states of agitation, insomnia, lack of appetite, functional epigastric disorders (nervous, irritable stomach, meteorism) and nervous intestinal problems.

Cultivation

Lavender needs light, permeable, slightly limy soil (ask at a garden store) in a sunny location—and that's all. Set the first—purchased—plants in May, about 16 inches (40 cm) apart, press the soil firmly around the roots, water copiously, and cover with a damp peat layer 1 to 1.5 inches (3–4 cm) deep.

Don't worry if the plants show only modest growth the first year and produce few blooms; that is normal. The next year, however, the flowering shoots will be prolific. After the lavender blooms, toward the end of August, cut back the lavender subshrubs by about one-half. In winter cover them with some peat moss or mulch or fir brush.

Harvest the lavender flowers just as they are opening, when the essential oil content is greatest and the fragrance purest. Cut off the flowering shoots, tie them into bundles, and hang them up to dry in a dust-free, well-ventilated place. This old method of preparation has proved most reliable, because the essential oil survives best in this way. Once the bunches are dry, strip off the flowers and store them protected from light and dampness.

Lemon Balm: Folk Medicine's Universal Remedy

Melissa officinalis is the botanical name for lemon balm plant, on which many common names have been bestowed: sweet balm, melissa, honey plant, dropsy plant, cure-all, and citronele.

Lemon balm, like many other medicinal plants that are rich in essential oils (for example, peppermint and thyme), belongs to the mint family (Lamiaceae = Labiatae). The original home of lemon balm is the Near East. From there it quickly found its way to Europe and across the Alps. It was the Benedictines who put it in their monastery gardens. In his capitulary on the management of the royal estates (*Capitulare de villis*), Charlemagne finally directed (about A.D. 810) that his subjects plant lemon balm throughout his domain. Today it continues to be grown in many gardens as a medicinal plant and for culinary use. Lemon balm is seldom found growing wild; the balm leaves used for pharmaceutical purposes are cultivated. Spanish balm, owing to its high essential oil content, has a special reputation.

Lemon balm is a profusely branching herbaceous plant that can reach 12 to 28 inches (30–70 cm) in height. It bears opposite leaves on square stems. White or whitish-yellow flowers form in false whorls at the axils of the leaves. The blooming season is during the months of July and August.

In folk medicine, lemon balm is considered a universal remedy, one to which one always resorts whenever health disturbances occur: in the gastrointestinal area, in the gallbladder or liver, in the heart, during menstruation, during menopause, or with illnesses caused by colds. Lemon balm often can be used with great success as a remedy for nervousness and sleep disturbances.

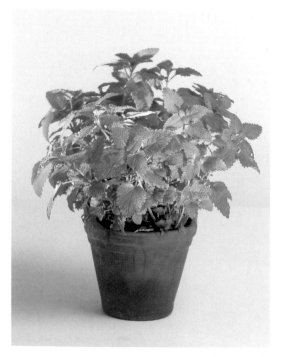

Lemon Balm

Scientists also have acknowledged lemon balm as an especially effective medicinal plant, whose calmative, spasmolytic, choleretic, aperitive, and carminative properties are well documented. In addition, the essential oil of the lemon balm plant (hence the tea infusion as well) prevents the spread of bacteria, viruses, and even fungi.

The German Office of Health lists the following areas of application for lemon balm leaves: Insomnia caused by nervous tension, gastrointestinal upsets, and lack of appetite.

Cultivation

This medicinal plant is one of the most popular medicinal herbs. It can be grown from seed, of course, but it is simpler to get some slips (divided plants) from friends or to buy some in a garden store. In early spring or in fall, set them in loosened soil spaced 14 to 16 inches (35–40 cm) apart. Tend the slips by shallowly hoeing up the ground, watering occasionally, and applying some mineral fertilizer. That is all that is required.

Lemon balm is a herbaceous plant that can live for many years. It has proved helpful, however, to separate and transplant the stems every three to five years; this ensures that the leaves will retain their full aroma.

If you have no garden, you also can grow lemon balm in pots on the balcony or patio; in this case, however, you will need to repot every fall or, preferably, set new cuttings.

For culinary purposes the fresh leaves are used; for making tea, use dried balm leaves harvested before the bloom. Cut the shoots off about 4 inches (10 cm) above the ground, tie them into bunches, and hang them up to dry in a well-ventilated place. After they are dry, strip the leaves off the stems, dry them again briefly (in your oven at about 95°F [35°C]), and store the drug in containers that can be tightly closed, protected from dampness and light.

Licorice: The Confection Is Made from It

There are two different areas of application, both acknowledged by the German Office of Health, for chopped or powdered licorice roots and the licorice extract made from them: loosening phlegm and making expectoration easier in catarrhs of the upper respiratory passages (bronchitis); supportive therapy in the treatment of cramplike disturbances in inflammations of the gastric mucosa (chronic gastritis).

Licorice is an important and valuable healing drug, but it is not without its problems.

Please note

The application of the tea or the licorice extract should continue for no more than four to six weeks; otherwise, increased retention of water can result, with swelling in the face and the ankle joints. People with liver disease, high blood pressure, and low levels of potassium in their blood must not use licorice.

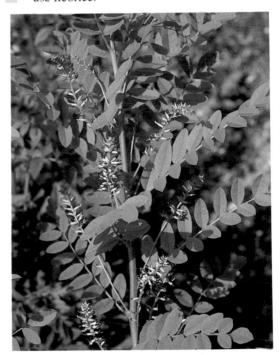

Licorice

Glycyrrhiza glabra is the botanical name of the licorice plant, which belongs to the bean family (Fabaceae = Leguminosae). It is native to the Mediterranean region, central and southern Russia, and Asia Minor as far as Iran. The healing drug comes almost exclusively from cultivation. *Glycyrrhiza lepidote*, a North American native species, may be substituted.

Licorice is a woody herbaceous perennial that grows 39 to 59 inches (1–1.5 m) tall. It has an extensive root system with a taproot, adventitious roots, and extremely long stolons. The leaves are imparipinnate, and the 9 to 17 pinnae are oval to heart-shaped and have short, abruptly projecting points. The racemes, with 20 to 30 pale-lilac papilionaceous flowers, arise from the leaf axils.

Cultivation

Raising licorice in your backyard garden is not recommended.

Linden

Among the Germanic peoples the linden was a "sacred" tree for people in love, the tree that brought fertility and prosperity. In the Middle Ages, people carved images of the Virgin Mary and figures of saints from linden wood, calling the wood *lignum sacrum*, sacred wood. Nothing is known to us from ancient times about the use of the linden flowers, which are so popular today. In ancient herbals or collections of writings no mention is made of linden flowers; even Abbess Hildegard of Bingen, who was skilled in medicine, writes only that the linden is quite salutary.

Today, however, linden flowers are prized as a preventive of colds. Head colds in particular usually can be warded off through prompt application of linden flower tea, along with a footbath. Linden flower tea also has proved effective against dry coughs, and people suffering from rheumatism drink the tea to ease their pain.

The German Office of Health recommends linden flowers to soothe the irritation in the

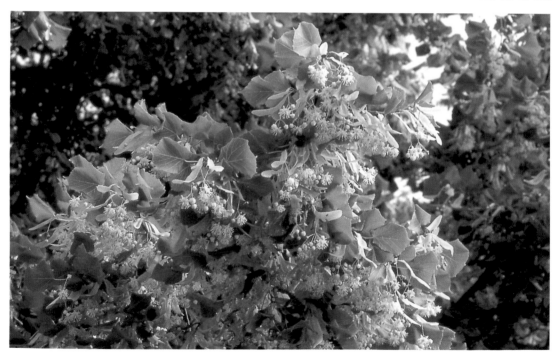

Linden

throat that causes coughing in catarrhs of the respiratory passages and in colds accompanied by fever, when a sweat cure is called for.

Naturopaths have discovered that charcoal made from linden wood, when taken in powdered form, alleviates symptoms of fermentation in the intestinal tract that are accompanied by foul-smelling diarrhea. The charcoal powder also can relax spasms in the colon.

It is probably unnecessary to describe the linden, for everyone knows this popular tree, a familiar sight in gardens, village squares, and parks. Far fewer people are aware, however, that there are two linden species that are used medicinally: the summer linden (*Tilia platyphyllos*) and the winter linden (*Tilia cordata*) family Tiliaceae. The winter linden blooms about two weeks earlier than the summer linden. The winter linden is smaller in stature and has smaller leaves, but its inflorescences bloom more abundantly. On the undersides of its leaves, reddish-yellow tufted hairs are located in the axils of the leaf veins. They are not present in the summer linden. Medicinal use is made of the inflorescences of both species, along with the adhering parchment-like bract. They are harvested shortly after the flowers have opened, because they yield the most effective tea in the first three days of bloom. After the harvest, the inflorescences have to be dried quickly. This can be done in the open air or in your kitchen oven, with the door open, at a temperature no higher than 104°F (40°C).

Keep the dried, chopped linden flowers in a container that can be tightly closed, protected from light and dampness, so that you will have a fragrant, effective house tea on hand at all times.

Cultivation

If you have a large yard and garden or, even better, a park to call your own, you ought to have a linden tree in it. Once you become familiar with the beneficial effect of the linden flower and the delicious taste of linden flower tea with honey, you will gladly harvest linden leaves year after year, despite the risk of bee stings. When the bees are buzzing around the garden, you know that the time has come to harvest the flowers. The linden flowers must be harvested within the first three to five days after they bloom, and this is precisely the period when the bees are busy too.

Very few people, however, have a large garden, much less a park. Quite recently, however, dwarf linden trees became available, and they will fit in any small garden. They bloom abundantly, and their flowers are just as valuable as those of the large linden tree.

The dwarf linden is happy in any garden soil. It needs sun, nothing more. Ask about a dwarf linden at a garden store or a nursery; it will enliven your garden and supply you with healthful linden flower tea.

Lingonberry (Mountain Cranberry): Popular Not Only as a Side Dish with Game

Wherever blueberries (see page 149) grow, you generally also will find lingonberries, though in far smaller numbers.

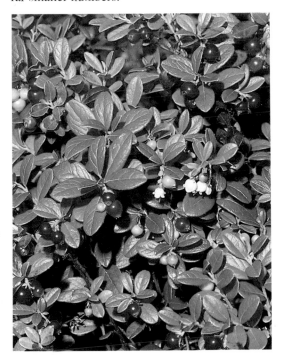

Lingonberry

Vaccinium vitis-idaea is the botanical name of this small subshrub, which, like the blueberry, belongs to the heath family (Ericaceae). Lingonberry lies close to the ground. Its leaves are leathery, obovate, and blunt at the tip, with involuted margins. The upper surfaces of the leaves are dark green, the undersides, pale green in color. The flowers, which occur in clusters, have a bell-shaped corolla 8 to 10 millimeters long. This flower head is up to 50 percent quinquefid, with pointed tips that curve outward. The spherical fruits are brilliant red.

At one time the leaves, like those of bearberry plants, were used as bladder and kidney remedies. Today, however, they are rarely used for that purpose, as the effect of bearberry leaves is far superior.

What makes the berries popular as more than a side dish with venison and other game, however, is the fact that little children who don't want to eat can be cured of their lack of appetite by 1 teaspoonful of lingonberry jam two or three times a day—and this medicine has no side effects.

Please note

To avoid mistaking bearberry (see page 143), which is quite similar in appearance, for lingonberry, you need to look at the underside of the leaf. The undersides of bearberry leaves never are dotted with brown, whereas lingonberry leaves always have minute brown dots below. I also want to point out that lingonberries should be harvested only when fully matured, because the ripening process will not continue during storage. The taste of unripe berries ranges from unpleasantly tart to bitter.

Cultivation

Lingonberries are unsuitable for raising in your backyard garden.

Madder: Once a Sought-after, Popular Dye

The trousers of the French soldiers of the nineteenth century and the head coverings of the Turks, the fezzes, once were dyed red with madder. This striking coloring agent held its own until aniline dyes came along. It is the roots that contain the red coloring—today we know that it is due to anthraquinone derivatives.

The madder plant, *Rubia tinctorum* L., better known as dyer's madder, is native to southern Europe and western Asia. Like sweet woodruff, it belongs to the madder family (Rubiaceae). Madder is a perennial herbaceous plant with decumbent or climbing square stems, which bear small lanceolate leaves and yellowish-green flowers. The rhizome, which creeps in the soil, grows over 39 inches (1 m) long. When dried and ground, it yielded the dye known as Turkish red. Madder is one of the oldest coloring agents known to us; it was used in pre-Christian times by the Egyptians, Persians, and Indians.

Like many other Mediterranean plants, madder was brought across the Alps by Benedictine monks, and Charlemagne, in his capitulary on the management of his landed estates, called for it to be grown within his domain.

The medicinal use of madder roots can be traced back to the adherents of Hippocrates in

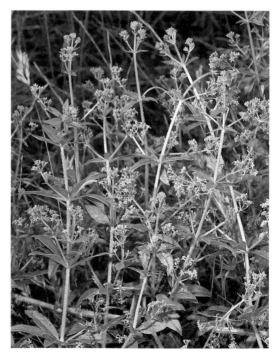

Madder

the fifth and fourth centuries B.C., who considered them an excellent antidiarrheal agent. They were used for that purpose until the second century A.D. Then, however, they were employed as remedies for such a multitude of different complaints and conditions that it is impossible to enumerate them all.

Today we use madder root, the tincture prepared from it, or a root extract to treat urinary calculus. In the course of the application, the dyes (derivatives of alizarin) pass into the urine, which thus acquires a red color. Patients treated with madder root must be given that information, lest they not interpret the red stained urine as "bloody urine." Ruberythric acid and its derivatives, viewed as the primary active substance of madder root, inhibit the precipitation of calcium phosphates and calcium oxalates and thus prevent the production of phosphate and oxalate stones. To dyer's madder is also attributed the power to reduce the size of urinary calculus by dissolving out the oxalates and phosphates: As a result of the drug's antispasmodic property, urinary calculus can be excreted more easily.

Madder now is seldom used as a tea, not least because it doesn't taste especially good. Taking the powder in capsules avoids the taste problem.

Cultivation
Raising madder yourself is possible but it usually becomes invasive in the garden.

Marjoram: Fragrant and Minty-smelling

From this medicinal plant, a traditional remedy for head colds—marjoram ointment, or salve—is prepared. It is particularly beneficial for infants and young children. In addition, marjoram is equally tasty and popular as a culinary herb, in which form I particularly commend it to older people. It ensures easy digestion even of fatty or flatulence-producing foods, stimulates the appetite, and makes an excellent seasoning for sauces, fried potatoes, and—in small amounts—salads as well.

In classical antiquity, marjoram, sacred to Aphrodite, was reputedly a means of arousing desire and bestowing potency. For these purposes it was added to wine.

Since the sixteenth century, marjoram has been known as a seasoning, and also as an herbal remedy for stomach and intestinal disorders. In particular, however, it is known as the base substance for the preparation of marjoram ointment, which, as I have stated, is effective against head colds and also—when rubbed into the area surrounding the navel—is a remedy for gas pains in infants.

Origanum majorana is the botanical name of marjoram, a member of the mint family (Lamiaceae = Labiatae). It is also known as sweet marjoram and wild marjoram. Oregano (*Origanum vulgaris*) is a closely related perennial. Native to peninsular India and naturalized in Arabia, Egypt, and the Mediterranean countries, it was unable to become established north of the Alps. In North America it is found principally in

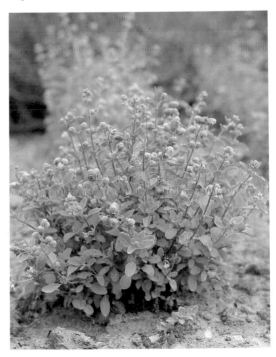

Marjoram

herb gardens, though it sometimes escapes from cultivation.

Marjoram reaches a height of 8 to 20 inches (20–50 cm), branches profusely, and grows erect. It has squared, slender, tough stems and branches, on which small spatulate, entire, rounded leaves grow. These leaves, which are hairy on both sides, also may grow on short stalks, in which case they are arranged in pairs on opposite sides of the stalk. The shoots are covered with downy hair and sometimes have a reddish tinge. The light-red or white labiate flowers occur in dense, egg-shaped false spikes at the axils of the bracts.

The entire plant has an aromatic smell. This scent and the spicy, pungent taste probably account for the popularity of marjoram.

Cultivation

Marjoram is an annual that has to be grown from seed. As it is extremely frost-tender, it is best to sow it in March in a cold frame. Only in May, after the last frost date is past, can it be set outdoors—spaced 6 inches (15 cm) apart in light, nutritious garden soil. Some plants also can be set in balcony planters or flowerpots. A sunny location, which also has to be protected from wind, is best for the plants. Because marjoram grows fairly slowly, you will have to be diligent about removing any nearby weeds to keep it from being overrun.

Shortly before the blooming season is the proper time for harvesting, because the content of aromatic substances is highest then. Cut down the herbs, tie them into bunches, dry them in the open air, and store them where they will stay dry and be protected from light (metal boxes are suitable).

Marshmallow: Used as a Medicinal Plant in Antiquity

Marshmallow, known to botanists as *Althaea officinalis*, is a member of the mallow family (Malvaceae). The medicinal effect of its roots has been known since antiquity; it is interesting that the same problems are treated with marshmallow tea today as in earlier times. The soothing effect is due to the high mucilage content of the roots. This plant mucilage forms a protective coating on the inflamed mucous membranes of the mouth and throat, as well as those of the stomach and intestinal tract. For this reason we use marshmallow tea to treat pharyngitis, sore throat, dry cough, hoarseness, and inflamed gastric and intestinal mucosae.

The German Office of Health acknowledges the medicinal effect of marshmallow roots, specifically their ability to soothe inflammations of the mucous membranes in the mouth and throat areas, the upper respiratory passages, and the stomach and intestinal canal.

At this point I want to mention again a special feature of the preparation of this tea. Marshmallow root tea has to be made with cold water. For this reason it is ill suited as a component of tea blends that are brewed with hot water.

Marshmallow originated in the countries surrounding the Caspian Sea, the Black Sea, and

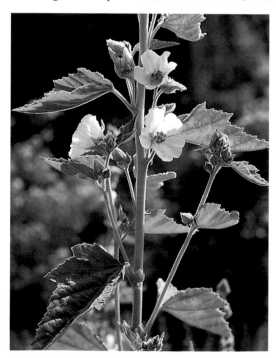

Marshmallow

the eastern Mediterranean. It became naturalized in North America, where several species are found in the wild. This hairy herbaceous perennial grows over 39 inches (1 m) tall. The leaves, whose stalks are arranged spirally on the stem, are covered with feltlike, whitish hair; they have three to five lobes, with irregularly crenate margins. In the leaf axils, stemmed flowers with white or reddish petals grow in clusters. The flowers bloom in June, July, and August.

Cultivation

In many places, marshmallow is known as "sweetwood." If you have some room along your garden fence, be sure to give it to this medicinal plant. You can grow marshmallow from seed, of course, but it is simpler to buy young plants and set them in June, spaced 12 to 16 inches (30–40 cm) apart. Marshmallow needs a sunny location with humus, deep, moist, but not heavy soil.

If you have a large balcony, you also can try raising marshmallow there, in a tub or an earthenware container (at least as large as a water pail). The prepared soil needs a high nitrogen content, and every two weeks more fertilizer has to be added along with the sprinkling water. Your garden store or a neighbor with experience can advise you.

By fall, the roots will be ready for harvesting, just in time to have marshmallow tea or marshmallow syrup on hand to combat winter coughs. When harvesting, cut off the aerial parts of the plant about 2 inches (5 cm) above the soil. Then, with a garden fork, dig out the rhizomes and cut off the young roots, which are the medicinally useful parts of the plant. The rhizome heads from which the young roots were removed can be sown again immediately.

Rinse the young roots briefly; cut them into either manageable pieces or smaller, "tea-sized," pieces and dry them thoroughly in a 131°F (55°C) oven. Then store them in a container with an airtight closure. Their greatest enemy during storage is moisture, as marshmallow's high starch content causes it to become moldy quickly if it gets damp.

Milk Thistle Fruits: Known as a Liver Protective

Since the silymarin complex contained in the milk thistle, or marian thistle, was studied more closely and it became known how great its ability is to protect the liver, this thistle has been very much in the limelight again. Thus the popularity of the fruits in the treatment of liver problems has some factual basis. Nevertheless, scientists are reserved in their recommendation of the tea made from these fruits, because very little silymarin finds its way into the tea. Consequently the German Office of Health endorses the use of this tea only for mild indigestion.

I think this conservative stance is exaggerated, because the drug has been used for centuries to treat liver disease, hepatitis, and fatty infiltration of the liver. For this reason I consider the fruits a valuable component of teas for liver, gallbladder, and gastrointestinal complaints as well as blood-purifying teas. Application in a proper course of treatment is important, however.

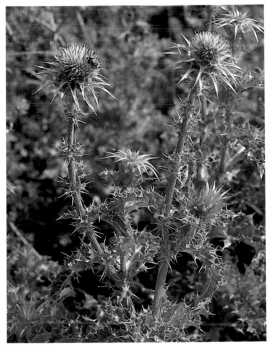

Milk Thistle

The milk thistle, *Silybum marianum* (= *Carduus marianus*), family Compositae = Asteraceae, is one of the most attractive thistles. It can be recognized easily by its large, greenish-white veined leaves, which have prickly edges. The small composite flowers, reddish-violet in color, are borne in solitary spherical heads at the ends of the stalks. From the fertilized inflorescences develop hard fruits with a silky crown of hair, which is soon shed, however. These fruits constitute the drug (milk thistle fruits). The milk thistle is native to southern Europe, southern Russia, Asia Minor, and North Africa. It is naturalized in America, and is grown in gardens as an ornamental.

Cultivation

If you have a large garden, you can "afford" to grow milk thistle. It is quite a beautiful plant, but it needs a great deal of room, as it can reach a height of over 6.5 feet (2 m). It is most practical to get one or several little seedlings from a garden store and set them in your garden in a

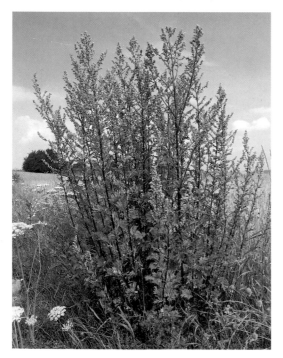

Mugwort

warm, dry spot. In good garden soil the plant will become quite luxuriant. It will bloom in late summer and also produce ripe fruits, which will self-sow and provide successors the following year. If you want to try, you can raise milk thistle in large tubs on your patio or balcony. Each plant needs its own tub. The seedlings should be set in spring. Warmth and scant moisture are the prerequisites for good growth.

Mugwort: The Milder, Gentler Brother of Wormwood

Mugwort is *Artemisia vulgaris* L., a member of the Compositae = Asteraceae family. Outwardly these two medicinal plants are extremely similar; they are used equally as medicinal plants and as seasonings. For this reason I refer you to the "Wormwood" profile on page 212. There you will find everything you need to know about mugwort—any differences from wormwood in appearance or application are described there, along with valuable information on raising it in your garden.

Worth mentioning: Many people are allergic to mugwort pollen from July to September.

Mullein: A Popular Cough Remedy Among the Ancient Greeks

Plants that look so stately and produce new flowers continuously for many weeks would naturally attract people's attention. The flowers were used successfully to treat colds, especially those accompanied by coughs. The cold-method extract in olive oil, the so-called king's oil, was esteemed as a vulnerary.

Mullein was in ancient times a magical plant, used in attempts to ward off lightning, disease, and dangers conjured up by evil spirits. At the time of Charlemagne it also was misused for catching fish in "forbidden" waters. If you boil down a large quantity of mullein plants in water and pour the decoction into fish ponds, the saponins in the mullein will reduce the surface tension of the water to such an extent that the water will get into the gills of the fish, which then drown in their own "element." Since Hildegard of Bingen praised mullein for its power to relieve chest and lung ailments, it has been valued as a cough remedy in Germany.

Today mullein flowers are an effective ingredient of various tea blends for treating coughs, especially those blends intended to loosen viscid mucus and facilitate its expulsion. The German Office of Health recommends mullein for colds and coughs, to soothe irritation and make expectoration easier.

Today we have to regard primarily the mucilage, the saponins, and the flavonoids, in addition to numerous other constituents, as active substances.

The two mullein species used for medicinal purposes are large-flowered mullein (*Verbascum thapsus* L.) and common mullein (*Verbascum phlomoides*), which belong to the snapdragon family (Scrophulariaceae). They often grow on slopes, railroad embankments, stony inclines, and waste land, and they can reach a height of

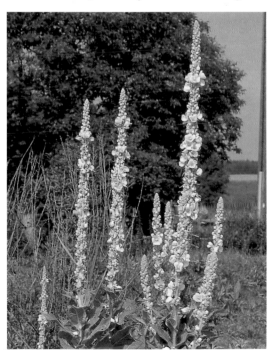

Mullein

over 6 feet (2 m). Golden-yellow flowers, united in bunches of two to five, grow densely along the long, sometimes diversely branching flowering stalks

Cultivation

You need plenty of space for mullein, as the plants can grow over 6 feet (2 m) tall. They are not difficult to raise. First get seed, which you sow in a garden bed in April or May. Leaf rosettes will form, and they need to be thinned out to a distance of about 4 inches (10 cm) apart. In fall, transplant them to the place where you want them to grow. The location has to be sunny and somewhat protected from wind. Mullein places no special demands on the soil; any garden soil will suit it.

The next year the flowering stalk will develop from the leaf rosette and grow to an imposing height. After the flowers fade, the shallow-rooted plants can simply be pulled out of the ground.

Once you have mullein in your garden and leave a plant standing until the seeds ripen, you need never worry about offspring. You will find leaf rosettes in every possible location, and you have only to transplant them to the places where you want mullein to grow.

Harvest the golden-yellow flowers only in good weather, if you want to ensure that the tea will retain its eye appeal. The best time for gathering is late morning, after the sun has dried the dew. Then the flowers can be picked easily. Only the corollas with the stamens that occur on them should be collected. They have to be dried without delay, ideally in your kitchen oven, with its door open, at a temperature of 122°F (50°C). When the flowers are thoroughly dry, put them immediately into containers that can be tightly closed. Because they are extraordinarily sensitive to dampness, you need to place a desiccant (yellow diatomaceous earth or self-indicating silica gel, available in pharmacies) in the storage container.

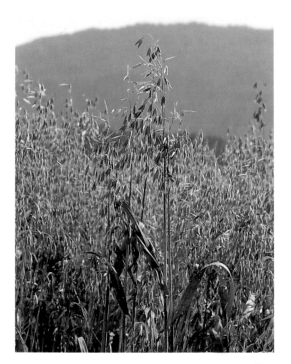

Oats

panicle, or compound raceme. The grains of oats that develop at maturity are surrounded by glumes, with which they are not fused. The blooming season is June to August, depending on the elevation. Oats can be raised at elevations of over .9 mile (1500 m).

Oats contain proteins; B vitamins; minerals such as phosphorus, iron, cobalt, manganese, zinc, aluminum, and potassium; vitamin K and vitamin E; provitamin A (carotene); and the trace elements boron and iodine. The silicic acid ought to be of interest for the use of oat straw as a bath. The calming effect of oats is due chiefly to avenine, an indole alkaloid. To take advantage of its calming effect, alcohol-based extracts from the oat kernels (grains) or the oat leaves and stems are used primarily, in addition to oat straw baths and tea made from the leaves and stems. You can make such an extract yourself, starting with oat kernels and 70 percent pure grain alcohol (vodka or undenatured ethyl alcohol, **not rubbing alcohol**) in a 1:10 ratio, but the homeopathic 1x, available in pharmacies under the name *Avena sativa* 1x, has been demonstrated to be superior to this extract. The homeopathic agent is made from fresh, flowering plants. To combat nervousness and agitation, take 5 drops several times a day. To use as a sedative, take 20 to 25 drops about one hour before bedtime.

Oats: Esteemed as a Medicinal Plant, Forgotten, and Rediscovered

When we hear the word "oats" today, we think of oatmeal porridge, gruel, and other dishes prepared from oats and used as part of a bland diet for innumerable ailments, a dietary food, or a means of strengthening debilitated patients. Only old country folk still know oats as a sedative, however. Oats once took the form of oat drops, oat tea, or oat baths. These applications are regaining importance today.

Oat, or *Avena sativa* (Poaceae = Gramineae family) by its botanical name, is a sweet grass grown everywhere in this country as a crop. Like all other cereals, oats grows erect and bears its flower at the end of a hollow stem. The flowers are arranged in panicles, or, more precisely: The spikes, which consist of two to four flowers, are borne on twigs, which on their part form the

Cultivation
Oats are not suitable for raising in a backyard garden.

Orthosiphon Leaves: Relative Newcomers to Europe

This plant, native to tropical Asia, has been known in Europe as a remedy for bladder and kidney complaints only since the 1920s. It was official in the Dutch Pharmacopoeia of 1926. Since that time it has become so popular, however, that the numbers of plants growing in the wild are no longer sufficient to satisfy the demand. For this reason, orthosiphon is cultivated in Indonesia, the source of most imports. It is

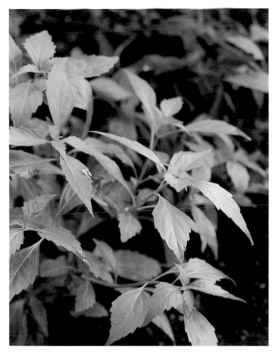

Orthosiphon leaves

the production of urine, in patients with catarrhs in the kidney and bladder area, for example.

The botanical name of orthosiphon leaves is *Orthosiphon spicatus*. This plant, a member of the mint family (Lamiaceae), can reach 39 inches (1 m) in height. It has a squared stem, on which the leaves grow in a decussate arrangement. The leaves, which grow 2 to 2.4 inches (5-6 cm) long and .4 to .8 inch (1–2 cm) wide, are short-stalked, ovate to lanceolate, and sharply pointed at the tip; they are not unlike peppermint leaves. At the shoot ends grow bluish-white labiate flowers in six-blossomed false whorls, joined to form an extended false spike, on short stems. The leaves and flowers have an aromatic smell.

Cultivation
Not suitable for raising in a backyard garden.

Pansy or Violet: For Young Girls with Blemished Skin

Our grandmother set great store by the wild violet or pansy. Innumerable times she recommended washes with the tea infusion: for blemished skin, psoriasis, acne, and infants' cradle cap. And the results were good. Every spring, when it was time to put together a tea blend for a spring tonic, a "blood-purifying cure," wild pansies had to be part of it—to benefit the skin. And then the tea was also believed to be a means of strengthening resistance and preventing colds.

In the monograph authored by Commission E of the German Office of Health, external application of pansy tea is acknowledged as helpful in mild, seborrheic (scaly) skin diseases and in the cradle cap that affects children. Flavonoids, salicylic acid, and plant mucilages, as well as saponins, are listed as active substances.

Viola tricolor L., the tiny wild, or field, violet or pansy that is part of the violet family (Violaceae), is the original plant used for this medicinal tea. The plant grows in fields, dry meadows, and garden plots. It reaches a height of 8 to 12 inches (20–30 cm) and produces a

difficult to obtain in North America, but may be available through mail order catalogs.

"Orthosiphon leaves" is the official name of the drug, but it is better known as "Indian bladder and kidney tea." It also is called Koemis koetjing.

Orthosiphon leaves are an ideal supplement for bearberry leaves in the treatment of bladder and kidney catarrhs, because they have, along with their disinfective property, a slightly diuretic effect, which bearberry leaves lack. In addition, orthosiphon leaves also can be prepared by the cold-water method.

Amazingly, orthosiphon leaves have been the subject of very little scientific study. They are known to contain essential oils (about 0.5 percent), flavones, and mineral salts, predominantly potassium salts (about 3 percent). It is not yet certain whether saponins are included among the active substances. Where the effect is concerned, however, there is unanimity. The German Office of Health recognizes orthosiphon leaves as a medicinal tea and recommends them to promote

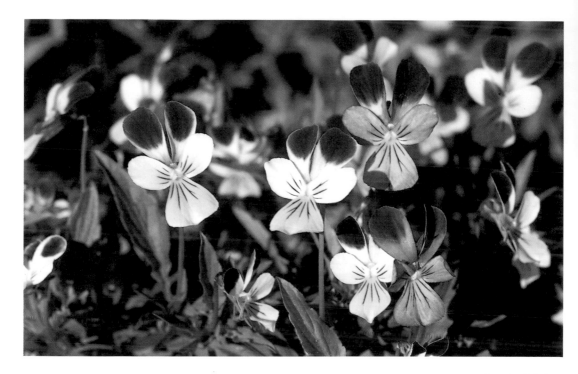

Pansies (Violets)

squarrose stalk on which lanceolate leaves grow. The flowers resemble those of our garden pansy; their colors range quite widely: yellow, blue, violet, or multicolored.

Cultivation

This flower is so common in meadows, fallow land, and fields that I advise against putting it in your herb garden, particularly as it does not grow very well there.

Passionflower (Maypops): A Healing Ornamental

It suddenly burst upon the medicinal plant market: the marvelously beautiful passionflower, *Passiflora incarnata*, a member of the Passifloraceae, a family botanically related to the violets. And indeed, this plant turned out to be a useful remedy for nervousness, sleep disturbances, and mild depression.

The passionflower is native to southern North America and Mexico; more than 400 different cultivars grow there. Many of them have fruits with juicy pulp, which are eaten as fruit and yield a delicious juice that is called passion juice. This refreshing juice is also said to possess an equalizing and relaxing effect.

For pharmaceutical purposes, the aerial parts of *Passiflora incarnata,* the flesh-colored passionflower plant, are used. The name of the plant was bestowed by a Jesuit, Padre Ferrari, who served as a missionary in Mexico. It was the unusual structure of the flowers in which he thought he saw the elements of the Crucifixion: The three stigmas were the three nails holding Christ to the cross, the five stamens were His wounds, and the fringed corona was His crown of thorns.

The passionflower, quite popular as an ornamental, produces long, bare, thin, slightly grooved climbing stems. The stalked, deeply trilobate, alternate leaves are wedge-shaped at the base. The leaf lobes are ovate to lanceolate, with tiny serrations along the margins. The leaf

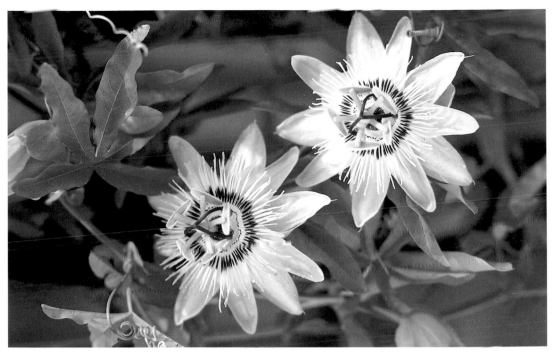

Passionflower (Mapops)

stalk has two extrafloral nectaries, or nectar glands. Long, single tendrils that contract tightly are produced in many leaf axils. The stalked flowers, which with their outspread sepals and petals measure about 3 inches (8 cm) across, occur in the axils of the leaves that are newest at the time. The sepals, which are cuspidate and oblong to ovate, grow together at their base to form a short tube. The petals are white, flesh-colored, or almost violet; they are shaped like the sepals, but are blunt, rather than cuspidate, at the tip. Within the petals is a dense fringed corona of purplish-red secondary petals, almost black toward the center. Passionflowers have five stamens and three stigmas, which coalesce at the base.

Passionflower is cultivated for pharmaceutical purposes. To obtain the tea drug, the aerial parts are collected during the blooming season and carefully dried. The homeopathic original tincture is prepared from the fresh aerial parts.

A tea made from the aerial parts of the passionflower plant is recognized, especially in the treatment of children, as a good remedy and palliative for nervousness, sleep disturbances, states of anxiety, and restlessness. Mixed with other calmative herbs (lemon balm, valerian, hop, St. John's wort), the aerial parts of passionflower are an effective ingredient of soporific teas and nerve teas.

Homeopathy uses *Passiflora* as an original tincture or in the lower potencies 1x or 2x to induce sleep.

Although the active substances of passionflower have been thoroughly studied, research does not conclusively indicate which of these components is the primary active substance.

Cultivation
Passionflower, which grows readily in southern California and Florida, can be cultivatd as a container plant; besides its medicinal properties, is a welcome aesthetic addition to any garden.

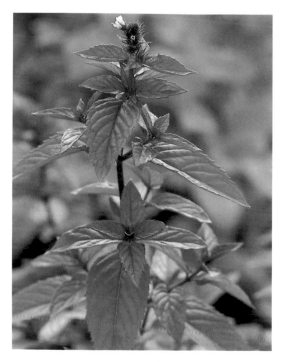

Peppermint

Peppermint: Among the Most Popular Remedies for Stomach, Intestinal, and Gallbladder Complaints

When queasiness, nausea, a feeling of fullness, or severe vomiting are the foremost problems, peppermint tea is the remedy of choice. With a single cup of peppermint tea, drunk in sips and as warm as possible, you can dispel these acute disturbances. Other gastrointestinal conditions such as flatulence, cramps, and diarrhea also vanish quickly and lastingly with therapeutic use of peppermint tea. If they do not, then the limits of self-medication have been reached. In such instances, consult a physician immediately, so that the precise cause of the problems can be brought to light.

Not least, however, peppermint tea promotes bile flow, improves bile production in the liver, and also exercises a positive influence on pancreatic function. Patients with gallstones enjoy drinking peppermint tea, but those with stomach ulcers cannot digest the tea especially well. Particularly when mixed with chamomile, peppermint is quite successful in the treatment of most gastric ulcers.

All these usages were not merely the therapeutic indications of folk medicine. Scientists also speak highly of peppermint. Under the heading "Areas of Application" the German Office of Health lists the following: Cramplike complaints in the gastrointestinal area, the gallbladder, and the bile ducts. And under the heading of "Effects": Direct spasmolytic (cramp-relieving) effect on the smooth muscles of the digestive tract; choleretic (stimulating bile production); carminative (causing the release of stomach or intestinal gas).

True peppermint, which botanists call *Mentha piperita*, is a member of the mint family (Lamiaceae = Labiatae). It is a cross (a hybrid) produced from spearmint (*Mentha spicata*) and water mint (*Mentha aquatica*). This hybrid appeared suddenly among the spearmint plants in a culture in England.

Mentha piperita grows almost 3 feet (90 cm) tall. Like all the other Labiatae, it has a square stem and decussate, ovate leaves. The whirled labiate flowers are whitish. The entire plant has a pleasant fragrance.

Cultivation

For raising in your garden, I recommend the English Mitcham peppermint, which tastes especially good.

Because crosses cannot be propagated by seed, you will have to get stolons from your garden store in spring. Soften the stolons in water for about two hours, then set them at least 8 inches (20 cm) apart in humus soil, in furrows about 2 inches (5 cm) deep. Initially you will need to water the slips daily, so that they will take root quickly. If it is to flourish, peppermint needs soil that is constantly damp—it does not tolerate prolonged dryness. If you loosen the soil occasionally, keep the plants free from weeds,

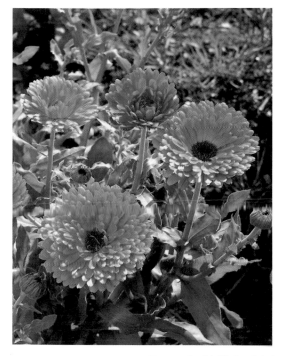

Pot marigold (Calendula)

popular plant is also known by the common name of pot marigold. It owes its German common name, *Ringelblume*, or ringed flower, to the simple fruits, which are closely curled almost in the shape of a ring at the center of the syncarps. The botanical name, *Calendula*, is derived from Latin *calendae*, meaning calends—the first day of the month in the ancient Roman calendar, as well as, by transference, a term for the month itself. We now assume that the name was intended to refer to the long blooming period of this medicinal plant, which flowers from May well into November.

Calendula flowers are relatively unimportant for internal use. A tea made from them is helpful in the treatment of gallbladder complaints, but more effective medicinal plants (peppermint leaves, the aerial parts of wormwood) are available for this purpose; it probably is included in the various tea blends more for cosmetic reasons than for its curative power. The golden-yellow petals look attractive in tea blends.

External application in the form of a compress prepared from the tea or of an ointment is quite helpful in treatment of poorly healing wounds, sprains, dislocations, strains, bloody effusions, and almost all "blunt" (not open) sports injuries. Lacerations, contusions, cuts, and burns heal painlessly and quickly if dressed with calendula ointment, and even infected wounds show improvement after treatment with the ointment.

The preventive and curative effects of calendula ointment in treating bedsores (decubitus ulcers) in bedridden patients was discovered—or perhaps rediscovered—in recent years.

The German Office of Health recognizes the healing effect of calendula. In the package enclosure, under "Application," it says this: Inflammations of the skin and mucous membranes; lacerations, contusions, and burns.

Calendula officinalis is an annual that reaches a height of about 20 to 28 inches (50–70 cm). The stem, covered with feltlike hair, is erect and branched. It bears alternate leaves, also covered with fine hair. The large, brilliant-yellow flower heads may measure over 1.6 inches (4 cm)

and fertilize a few times with compost, you will have performed all the care required. In winter, cover the plants with pine brush to protect them from cold.

Every three to five years you will have to transplant your peppermint plants to prevent backcrossing, which would cause them to lose their fragrance and their delicious taste.

To season foods, harvest fresh leaves as needed. Gather leaves for tea supplies shortly before the plants are due to bloom. For tea, pluck the leaves and dry them in a well-ventilated place or in your oven at 86 to 95°F (30–35°C). Then store them in a cool place, protected from light and dampness.

Pot Marigold (Calendula): Helpful with Wounds that Are Slow to Heal

You may be acquainted with calendula, *Calendula officinalis,* a member of the composite family (Asteraceae = Compositae). This

across. Calendula is native to central, eastern, and southern Europe.

Cultivation

Calendulas belong in every garden, if only for ornamental purposes, because their lengthy blooming season ensures enjoyment for a long while. There are different varieties, so if you want to use this medicinal plant for pharmaceutical purposes as well, be sure to choose the plant known as *Calendula officinalis*, and get the yellow-flowering variety. The seed is sown in early April in prepared beds, in rows spaced about 10 to 12 inches (25–30 cm) apart. Any good, slightly loamy garden soil is suitable. The location should be sunny. After two to three weeks the delicate little plants will appear. Water them assiduously, but avoid standing water.

For medicinal purposes, the parts used are the golden-yellow ligulate flowers, which should be plucked from fully opened flowers and quickly dried in a 122°F (50°C) oven with its door open. In storage the drug has to be protected from light and dampness.

Rose Hips: The Vitamin-rich Fruits of the Dog Rose

The dog rose, also called the dog brier or wild brier, is known to botanists as *Rosa canina* L. It is the original form of the numerous and diverse cultivated roses, whose flowers usually are double and have an intoxicating fragrance.

How modest this wild rose seems by contrast. It grows as a small shrub along the edges of woods and fields, in thickets and hedges, preferably on sunny heathland slopes and embankments. Rarely does it grow more than about 8 feet (2.5 m) tall. The small stems and branches droop. They bear imparipinnate leaves, which at their base are winged on both sides and consist of five to seven pinnules. The pale-pink flowers, which open in June and often in July as well, are single and odorless. The rose hips, which are brilliant red when ripe, develop from the fleshy floral axis. They contain numerous indehiscent fruits (achenes) as hard as stone and equipped with bristles—commonly known as "itching powder."

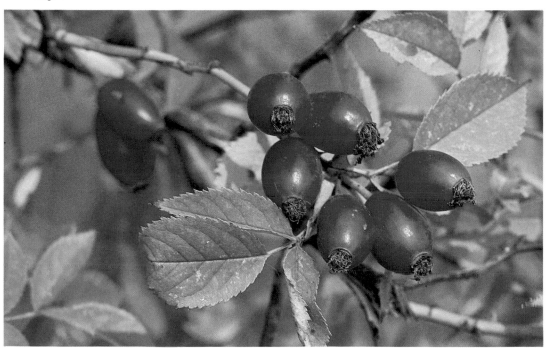

Rose Hips

For medicinal purposes, the parts used are the rose hips, because they have a refreshing taste and contain vitamin C, other vitamins and important minerals and trace elements. A tea prepared from the chopped, dried fruits makes an invigorating breakfast drink and is equally good as a thirst-quencher in summer and a hot beverage in winter. Rose hips are an ingredient of many tea blends, especially those drunk during cold season to prevent or alleviate flulike infections. Proof of specific effects has not been furnished thus far, apart from the mildly laxative action of the fruit acids or the slight diuretic action of the seeds in particular.

Also popular is a jam made from the overripe rose hips; it is said to stimulate the appetite and get those who are "not morning people" going. In Northern Bavaria, where it is known as rose hip pulp, it is used as a filling for pancakes.

Tea lovers who like to collect and prepare their medicinal plants themselves ask repeatedly whether they also can use other rose fruits for making tea infusions. In principle that is quite possible, but I advise against using the fruits of scented roses because allergic reactions have been observed in some instances.

The fruit of the potato rose, however, can be used to make a delicious tea. Because these fruits are quite juicy, however, drying them is difficult. They have to be dried in a 113°F (45°C) oven with its door open. In any event, dried rose hips need to be protected from light and dampness during storage.

Cultivation

If you have a large yard or garden, you need have no worry about planting several wild rose shrubs, which are available in nurseries. They need a sunny location and loamy, humus soil. They should not be planted until October or even November. Good watering is important; then the plants have to be "hilled"; that is, earth has to be heaped up around them. If you have no garden, you can also grow wild roses in tubs on your patio or balcony.

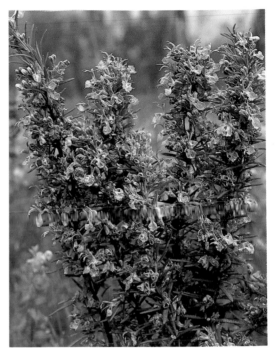

Rosemary

Rosemary: Almost a Universal Remedy in Medieval Times

In the first century A.D. Benedictine monks brought rosemary across the Alps from the warm Mediterranean countries, where it grows in abundance on dry slopes. Because it is not winter-hardy, it seldom succeeds in finding a home in the gardens north of Florida and southern California, but it is frequently grown in flowerpots.

Rosemary (*Rosmarinus officinalis* L.) a stately shrub with an aromatic smell, can reach a height of over 6 feet (2 m). Its profusely branched limbs are squarrose and densely covered with leathery, needlelike leaves with down-turned edges. The leaves are shiny above and covered with feltlike hair below. During the blooming season, which lasts from March until May, rosemary produces pale-blue, relatively small flowers, which are arranged in false whorls on the upper parts of the branches. A rich source of nectar, they are frequently visited by bees.

Through centuries of transmission from generation to generation, rosemary already had found a firm place in the herbals of the Middle Ages. Then when Pastor Sebastian Kneipp also gave his "blessing" to this medicinal plant, it dominated folk medicine through an extensive list of therapeutic indications. Preparations such as tea, wine, baths, and spirit were used in treating flatulence, gastrointestinal disturbances, lack of appetite, diseases of the pelvic organs, kidney, gallbladder, and liver complaints, edema, cardiac and circulatory problems, rheumatism and gout, cramps, paralysis, and, above all, nervous exhaustion. It also was used to strengthen convalescents.

For pharmaceutical purposes, the parts of rosemary used are the leaves. They contain essential oil, some saponin, and organic acids. The essential oil contains a substance that closely resembles the camphor found in the camphor tree; it is called rosemary camphor. This substance gives rosemary its tonic effect on the circulatory system and its equalizing effect on the nervous system. Rosemary is effective in all states of chronic debility, especially low blood pressure.

Rosemary wine, which you can make yourself, is quite popular: Pour 3/4 quart (3/4 L) of light Moselle wine over .35 to .70 ounces (10–20 g) of rosemary leaves in a wine bottle, let rest for five days, then strain. One small glass of wine twice a day is the proper dose.

An invigorating rosemary bath or—to stimulate circulation—a massage using spirit of rosemary are convincing in their effect. The preparations made from this medicinal plant are available in ready-to-use form in some pharmacies and health food stores.

Please note
Rosemary oil, which is the basis for the production of the spirit, may not be taken internally, as it irritates the stomach, intestinal tract, and kidneys.

Rosemary is also a delicious culinary herb, which you can add sparingly to all vegetable dishes. The taste of boiled fish, the gravy for the Sunday roast, and dishes containing poultry or mushrooms are also improved by the addition of rosemary. This seasoning also goes well with cheese; when mixed with rosemary (and thyme), every soft cheese becomes more easily digestible and more delicious. The following mixture of herbs and spices is recommended for anyone who enjoys highly seasoned food: equal parts of salt, pepper, thyme, rosemary, and cayenne pepper.

The German Office of Health recommends rosemary tea for people with a feeling of fullness, gas pains, and mild cramplike gastrointestinal disturbances and—applied externally—as a supplementary treatment for muscular and articular rheumatism.

Please note
Pregnant women should not drink the tea.

Cultivation
In areas where winters are extremely mild, rosemary can be grown outdoors year-round. However, it is difficult to grow rosemary in your garden in cooler regions. I recommend that you treat yourself to a vigorous rosemary plant at the garden store and put it in a large pot or tub. Fill the container with loose garden soil mixed with some peat and coarse sand. If you water the plant from time to time and put it in a sunny spot on your patio or in the yard, it will grow marvelously well. In winter bring it indoors, place it in a moderately warm spot (46 to 50°F [8– 10°C)—it has to be bright, however—and water it very scantly. Sometime in May the plant can be returned to the yard or the patio. Rosemary needs to be repotted and fertilized every other year.

Sage: A Versatile Medicinal Plant

"From now to all eternity you will be a favorite flower of mankind. I give you the power to heal men of all disease. Save them from death as you have done unto me." Thus, according to legend, the Virgin Mary spoke to the sage plant after it offered her a place to hide from the pursuit of Herod's men.

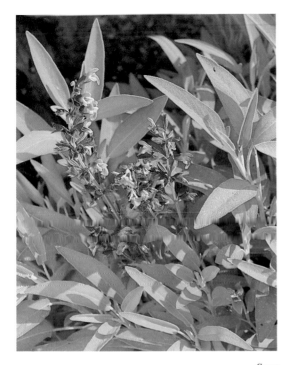

Sage

Salvia officinalis is the botanical name of true sage, a member of the mint family (Lamiaceae = Labiatae). Sage is native to the Mediterranean area, where it grows predominantly on mountain slopes, but now it is also widely cultivated. In its native habitat, the leaves also are prized, both as a pharmaceutical remedy (sage tea) and as a culinary herb.

True sage grows up to about 28 inches (70 cm) high. It is a subshrub with square stems covered with feltlike hair. The hairy elliptical, oblong, or ovate stalked leaves grow in opposite pairs on the stems. The light-blue to violet-blue flowers are arranged in loose racemes at the ends of the stems and branches.

Meadow sage, *Salvia pratense*, is not used for pharmaceutical purposes, but farmers feed this plant to pigs that are suffering from diarrhea, with a good rate of success.

If you have sage in your garden, make frequent use of the fresh leaves as a seasoning. They are good in ground meat, sausages, stews, and vegetable dishes and in stuffings for roasts. Chicken liver with sage is a favorite, and Saltimbocca alla romana is unimaginable without sage.

Put several spoonfuls of minced sage leaves in milk, bring it briefly to a boil, and serve it as a soup: This reputedly will build up the resistance of "sickly" children.

And truly: To this day sage continues to be a popular medicinal plant. In folk medicine the therapeutic indications are innumerable. It is used for gastrointestinal problems, diarrhea, liver disease, retention of bile, and circulatory disturbances. It also is used as an aid in weaning and to combat water retention, relieve colds, and treat inflammations of the mouth, throat, gums, and jaw. And that is by no means all.

Scientists are more reserved, of course, in their assessment of the powers of sage, but the spectrum of application is still amazingly large.

The German Office of Health recommends sage for inflammations of the gums and the mucous membranes of the mouth and throat; for pressure sores caused by dentures; as supportive therapy for stomach and intestinal catarrhs; and as a means to reduce elevated levels of secretion of sweat and saliva.

Responsible for the effect are the essential oil, tannins, bitter constituents, and flavonoids.

Cultivation

Equally popular as a culinary herb and a medicinal herb, sage made its conquest of our herb gardens long ago.

For your garden it is best to get several young plants and set them in April, spacing them about 16 inches (40 cm) apart, in normal garden soil. The location should be sunny or partially sunny, but protected from the wind. Thorough watering is necessary in prolonged dry spells. Loosening the soil and weeding are the only other tending required. As with peppermint, lemon balm, and thyme, it is advisable to separate the stems every three years and transplant them, so that the leaves retain their aroma.

To keep frost from damaging the sage plants in winter, cover them in fall with pine branches. Cut the plants back in spring, removing just under half of the length of the aerial parts.

Sage also can be grown in containers on your balcony, provided that you supply enough minerals in the form of liquid fertilizer every spring. After three years you need to replace the plants.

Fresh leaves make a good potherb for culinary use; dried leaves are used for the medicinal tea. Harvest the leaves just before the flowers bloom, dry them in a 95°F (35°C) oven with its door open, and preserve them, protected from light and damp, in containers that can be tightly closed.

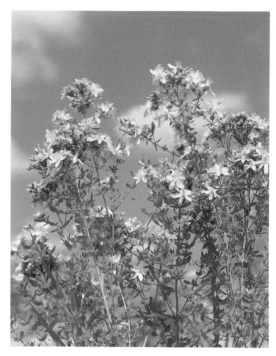

St. John's Wort

St. John's Wort: An "Herbal Tranquilizer"

We have to be slightly cautious with the term "St. John's wort," because many medicinal plants that flower about June 24 (St. John's Day) are called "St. John's wort." True St. John's wort, the plant used pharmaceutically, is *Hypericum perforatum*, commonly known also as amber touch-and-heal, goatweed, and rosin rose.

The botanical genus name, *Hypericum*, probably is derived from the Greek words hyper = over and eikon = image, intended to convey the belief that this plant is also effective against ghosts and spooks. Since at least the time of Paracelsus (1493–1541), we know, the plant was used to combat anxieties and bad dreams: " . . . for every physician should know that God has placed a great secret and powerful remedy in the herb, solely on account of the spectral and frightful fantasies that drive men to despair, and not through the devil, but through nature." (Paracelsus in the *Book of Original Things*, from about 1525).

True St. John's wort is common along roadsides, embankments, and field boundaries and in sparse woods and undergrowth. It is a herbaceous plant that grows about 10 to 36 inches (25–90 cm) tall. In its upper part, the stems branch profusely. The opposite leaves, which are elliptical, entire, and bare, range in size from .6 to 1.2 inches (1.5–3 cm). The golden-yellow flowers have five petals and are covered with blackish-red glandular scales.

True St. John's wort has three extraordinary features that help identify it and virtually rule out any possibility of mistaken identity: The stalk is two-edged, which is extremely rare in the plant kingdom. If you hold the leaves up to the light, you will see transparent dots (oil glands) on them that make the plant seem to be perforated; hence the species name *perforatum* and another of the English common names, hundred holes. The golden-yellow flowers turn dark red if rubbed between your fingers.

Originally St. John's wort, in the form of an oily extract, was used to treat skin damage (stab thrusts, injuries that were slow to heal). This too goes back to Paracelsus, who, in accordance with his doctrine of signatures, saw the "finger of God" in the oil glands of the leaves. Folk medicine also uses the oil of St. John's wort for pain caused by shingles and gout and for furunculosis and other ulcers and swellings.

Today it is the tea that ranks first in the pharmaceutical use of St. John's wort. Since the discovery was made that it can have a beneficial influence on mild depression, as well as on stress reactions and sleep disturbances, it has been in frequent use. After a four to six-week course of treatment with tea, a brightening of the patient's spirits is noticeable; peace and calm make an appearance, and falling asleep and staying asleep are no longer problematic. For these reasons, St. John's wort is added to the various teas used as sedatives, nerve tonics, and soporifics, as well as to teas for people with cardiac and circulatory conditions. Scientists acknowledge the value of true St. John's wort as a sedative and mild antidepressive. Calling it an herbal "tranquilizer," they ascribe this effect to the hypericin and other similar substances contained in the plant.

Please note
A side effect of this medicinal plant also has to be mentioned, however. After prolonged tea therapy, fair-skinned, sandy-haired people in particular suffer skin damage that resembles a sunburn. The burns result when the hypericin reacts with the light of sunlight, ultraviolet lamps, or tanning salons.

Cultivation
I really wonder why more people don't put this medicinal plant in their gardens. The golden-yellow flowers, which are profuse on the upper part of the plant, make St. John's wort a valuable addition to your garden. Moreover, it needs little care, and it is not at all demanding in terms of the soil it needs: limy, moderately heavy soil is perfectly suitable. This plant, however, requires plenty of sun. If you wanted to make things easy for yourself, you could bring several plants home from walks to set in your garden. Because we don't want to "plunder" nature, however,

you should grow St. John's wort from seed, as there is no objection to collecting the seeds of plants growing in the wild. When the seeds are ripe and can be easily shaken loose from the capsules, collect enough to fill a thimble. At home, dry them well and store them until the following spring. The tiny seeds will retain their germinating power for three years.

In May, sow the seed in small boxes of light garden soil and keep it moderately damp. After 14 to 20 days the seeds will germinate, and after another 14 days you can thin out the little plants. Two to three weeks later the seedlings will be ready for transplanting to a well-prepared garden bed (loosen the soil well) in a sunny location. Leave about 2.4 inches (6 cm) on all sides. In September the plants can be moved to their permanent location in the garden, where they should be set 8 inches (20 cm) apart on all sides. Then you need not worry further about them. The plants will survive even the coldest winter if covered with some brush. The following year the home-grown herbs will bloom. Then you can leave them alone, harvesting whatever you need, because St. John's wort is a herbaceous perennial.

Senna: Gentle, But Prompt Action

We are familiar with two species of senna that provide leaves and fruits for pharmaceutical use: *Cassia angustifolia*, also called Tinnevelly senna, is native to Somalia and Arabia and is cultivated primarily in the southern Indian district of Tinnevelly, to which it owes its name. *Cassia senna*, also known as Alexandria senna, is native to the Sudan and West Africa; it is cultivated primarily in the Upper Nile region.

Senna leaves and fruits are among the best-known laxatives: When an acute case of constipation needs to be remedied, or when a soft bowel movement is necessary after surgery in the anal area or as a result of other medical procedures, then these are the remedies of choice.

The German Office of Health recommends senna leaves and fruits in the treatment of all diseases in which a mild bowel movement with

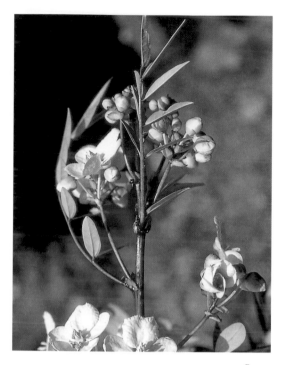

Senna

Please note
Without consultation with your physician, you should take senna leaves and fruits for only a short time! Do not use them in cases of intestinal obstruction!

Cultivation

Raising senna in your backyard garden is possible only in the Mediterranean and subtropical regions of North America. In cooler regions, it can be grown as a container plant. Water abundantly during the growing period and feed weekly until the end of August. Place the tub in full sun.

Sloe or Blackthorn: The Fruits Help Those Who Are "Not Morning People"

When the first frost of autumn has made its way through the country and when the kale has been harvested, it is time to pick sloe plums. Only then can their taste be "managed." True, they still taste tart and sour, but less so than in September, for example. These fruits are used to make jam or stewed fruit. according to the standard recipes for berries of all kinds, and this "medication" will help people who are not hungry in the morning, who usually go off to school or to work without having eaten a bite, which is certainly not advisable. Two to four spoonfuls of this jam, eaten before getting out of bed, are enough to enable someone to eat breakfast with a good appetite after about half an hour.

The sloe flowers, along with the young leaves, are still used in some places as a diuretic.

Prunus spinosa is the botanical name of the sloe, which is a member of the rose family (Rosaceae). It is a shrub growing about 3.3 feet to almost 10 feet (1–3 m) tall. Its branches, when young, are covered with velvety hair and end in sharp thorns. The stalked elliptical leaves have serrate edges. Even before the leaves unfold, the white, delicate flowers open, in such dense masses that the entire shrub is covered in white. From the flowers develop the berries, which at first are green, then dark blue, and later

a soft stool is desirable: with anal fissures and hemorrhoids and after rectal surgery; for cleaning the intestinal tract before x-ray examinations; and before and after surgery in the abdominal area.

Both species of senna are small shrubs 20 to 39 inches (50 cm–1 m) tall. They are papilionaceous plants (Fabaceae = Leguminosae), as are our common beans. The flattened brown fruits, .4 to .8 inch (1–2 cm) wide and .8 to 1.6 inches (2–4 cm) long, develop from the axillary yellow flowers, which grow in racemes. The fruits are known as "mother leaves" or "senna seedpods." When the leaves (pinnae) are fully developed, they are harvested by stripping, then dried in the open air. Do not harvest the fruits until they have matured fully.

For pharmaceutical purposes, it makes no difference which species the senna leaves come from; both are equally effective. The senna seedpods, however, should be those of Tinnevelly senna.

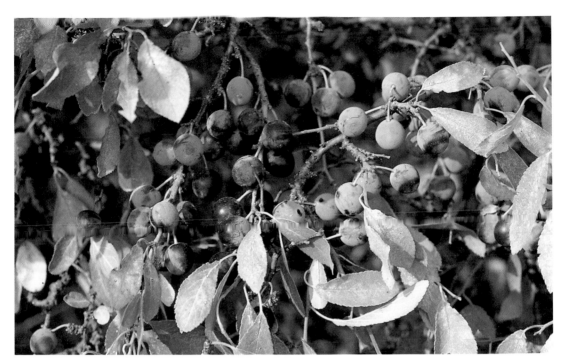

Sloe or Blackthorn

are covered with a frostlike bloom. They measure .4 inch (1 cm) in diameter.

Sloes are often found on sunny mountain slopes, along roadsides, at the edges of forests, on heaths, and in pastures, provided that enough lime is present in the soil.

Cultivation

Sloe makes an especially good live hedge in a garden. For this purpose, you need four to five bushes per 39 inches (1 m). They are available in garden stores. The soil has to be limy, permeable, and sandy to stony and loamy. Once the plants have struck root, they need no further care. You can let them grow in treelike shapes or trim them regularly.

Sloes also will grow in large tubs. The tub should be at least 18 inches (45 cm) deep and equally wide. Compost soil with some coarse sand and 1.76 ounces (50 g) of compound fertilizer per 2.6 gallons (10 L) of soil is the recommended soil for planting or repotting. A sloe growing in a trough planter needs to be repotted every other year in spring.

Stinging Nettle: Despised as a Weed—Prized as a Medicinal Herb

I can't imagine that there are people who have never been "stung" by a stinging nettle, for the lesser nettle (*Urtica urens*) and the common nettle (*Urtica dioica*) are extremely widespread—in gardens, in landfills, along fences and hedges.

Only the two commonly occurring species are used medicinally, however. Specifically, it is their leaves (or all the aerial parts) and roots that are used. The German Office of Health is extremely reserved in its assessment of this medicinal plant. It confirms that the stinging nettle is suitable for stimulating increased urine production and for supporting the treatment of problems in voiding urine.

Please note

Stinging nettle should not be used with edema (excessive accumulation of fluids) that is caused by reduced cardiac and renal activity.

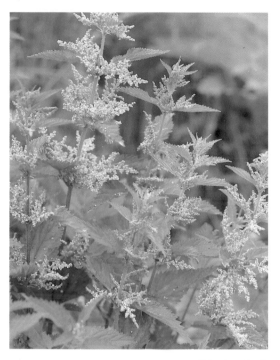

Stinging Nettle

Cultivation

Stinging nettle plants need not be specially culti-vated; they thrive everywhere they are allowed to grow. They are considered weeds, unwanted in vegetable gardens, orchards, or flower gar-dens; but wherever you make compost, next to the fence or in a corner of your orchard, you should let stinging nettles grow. Every year they can contribute their healthful leaves to enrich your spring salads; in summer you can harvest the leaves for a depurative tea; and in fall you can dig up the roots to turn into a tea drug as well: Wash them briefly, cut them into small pieces, and dry them in your oven at about 122°F (50°C).

If you leave stinging nettles standing here and there throughout your garden, you will not only do yourself a favor, but also preserve a food plant for several butterfly species.

Summer Savory: Both a Seasoning and a Medicinal Plant

With summer savory, as with basil, one is justi-fied in asking whether it is primarily a potherb or a medicinal plant; again, the answer is that it is equally important as both. In folk medicine it is used to treat gastric and intestinal complaints that are accompanied by fetid stools. I recom-mend it as a seasoning that stimulates the appetite and improves digestion, especially for use in the diets of older people, who can benefit their health greatly by proper consumption of hearty seasonings.

Basil, thyme, and summer savory, together with a little rosemary, can replace salt in our foods to a substantial degree. Summer savory goes well with all fatty roasted meats, including pork, duck, and goose, and with meat loaf. It adds interest to fried potatoes and is an excellent seasoning for sausage. For this reason, in many places it is also known as sausage herb.

Satureja hortensis is the botanical name of this member of the mint family (Lamiaceae = Labiatae). It probably originated in the regions around the Black Sea and the eastern

To that I would like to add that stinging nettle is also used successfully to purify the blood, to eliminate skin blemishes, and to treat rheuma-tism in the broadest sense. This is confirmed by physicians experienced in naturopathy.

A stinging nettle switch is recommended, for example, by Professor R. F. Weiss as an effec-tive remedy for sciatica and lumbago. First, tie stinging nettle (*Urtica dioica* is more practical) into a bundle to use as a switch, then scourge yourself with it, applying it to the painful areas of your body and the surrounding areas. After consulting with your physician, this treatment may be carried out for three days in succession, once each day. After an interval of three days, the procedure may be repeated.

Stinging nettle seeds reportedly have a tonic effect on older people, and the juice of stinging nettles is said not only to cleanse the blood, but also to have a beneficially stimulating effect on the pancreas. Neither the leaves nor the roots of stinging nettles—despite frequent claims to the contrary—are effective remedies for diabetes.

required. If the individual plants are too crowded, thin out the rows.

Winter savory (*Satureja montana*) has two subspecies, a decumbent form and an upright form. The subspecies are of equal value as potherbs. They also are propagated by seed, which, however, has to be sown in April in a cold frame. In May, set the seedlings in the ground outdoors, where they will last for five to six years. The soil should be loose and limy.

Fresh savory can be harvested all summer long and well into fall, with preference given to the flowers and leaves. For a winter supply, cut the plants a handsbreadth above ground level shortly before they are due to bloom, make bunches of them, and hang them up to dry. Store them where light and dampness cannot reach them.

Thyme: A Proven Remedy for Whooping Cough

Thymus vulgaris, true thyme, is native to the rocky heathlands and evergreen scrub of the Mediterranean area. Like a great many other medicinal plants from this region, it was brought across the Alps to monastery gardens by Benedictine monks. That must have occurred in about the eleventh century—quite late, when you consider that thyme has been used as a culinary herb and a medicinal plant for over 4000 years. Writings in Sumerian cuneiform from about 2000 B.C. tell us that in what presently is Iraq, thyme was grown, along with dill and coriander.

Today this herbaceous plant is grown in many backyard gardens. It also is cultivated commercially on a large scale for medicinal and culinary purposes. In addition to *Thymus vulgaris, Thymus zygis*—Spanish thyme—also has attained importance. The major components of the essential oil of thyme—thymol and carvacrol—are characterized by a rather strong disinfectant effect, and for this reason the medicinal plant is also used for gastrointestinal complaints that are accompanied by foul-smelling

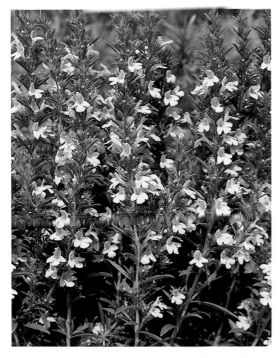

Summer Savory

Mediterranean. Benedictine monks brought it, along with many other potherbs, across the Alps to us, and Charlemagne, in his Capitulary on the management of his landed estates, ensured that it found its way into the gardens of monasteries and peasants' farms.

Satureja hortensis, an herb 12 to 16 inches (30–40 cm) tall, branches profusely from the ground up and produces lanceolate, pointed leaves on more or less hairy stems. Lilac to white flowers are borne in the leaf axils.

Cultivation

Two species are suitable for raising in your garden, the annual common summer savory and the perennial winter savory, also known as mountain savory. Common summer savory (*Satureja hortensis*) is sown in April in loose soil, in a warm location, at intervals of 10 inches (25 cm). Cover the seed loosely with soil. The seed will germinate in two or three weeks. Hoeing and weeding, along with occasional watering if no rain falls for some time, are the only care

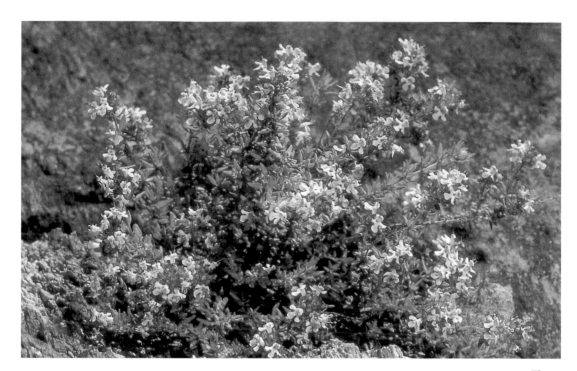

Thyme

stools and intestinal gases. Chiefly, however, thyme tea (and thyme baths also) is valued for its power to help those suffering from coughs and bronchial catarrhs, asthma and silicosis, and, above all, dry coughs and spasmodic coughs, as well as whooping cough in children. When a tickle in your throat announces the onset of a cold, you can nip it in the bud by gargling with thyme tea. The hot vapors of thyme tea also can be inhaled to relieve coughs, head colds, and frontal sinusitis.

It should be sufficiently well-known that thyme is a healthful flavoring. It makes all fatty roasts, including roast duck and roast goose, tastier and more easily digestible.

Thyme, a small subshrub of the mint family (Lamiaceae = Labiatae), grows up to 16 inches (40 cm) tall. The square stems are covered with short hairs and with leaflets only a few millimeters long. The pale-reddish typical labiate flowers occur in spikes. The entire plant is highly aromatic. All the aerial parts are harvested during the blooming season, which lasts from June to August. In harvesting, give preference to the shoot tips. High-quality products consist exclusively of the leaflets, stripped from the stem, and the flowers, without the lignified portions of the stems.

Cultivation

Two types of thyme, summer thyme and winter thyme, are available for culinary and medicinal herb gardens. In cooler latitudes it is necessary to choose the winter thyme, which is less demanding. In dry soil and in a warm, sunny location it will grow extremely well. Its ability to be content with very little is traceable to its origin, as its native habitat is the dry, warm Mediterranean area, where the soil is poor.

Regular hoeing up of the ground and weeding are the only tasks you need to perform to enable thyme to thrive. If the soil in your garden is very heavy, I recommend that you "loosen it up" with peat, sand, and some compost soil—ask for advice at a garden store.

Thyme is easiest to grow from herbaceous plants. It is best to get plants that are already full-grown from a garden store. Every three to five years, divide, cut back, and transplant the herbaceous plants.

For both pharmaceutical and culinary purposes, harvest thyme during the blooming season. Cut off the shoot tips, dry them in the open air or in artificial heat (not exceeding 95°F [35°C]), strip the leaves and flowers from the dried shoots, and store them in containers that can be tightly closed (see page 12).

Valerian. For Restful Sleep

We know valerian as an effective calmative for nervousness, a means to promote sleep, and a remedy for an overstrained heart. That was not always the case: At the time of Hippocrates (fifth to fourth centuries B.C.), valerian was used chiefly for gynecological complaints. In the Middle Ages new ranges of application were added: Hildegard of Bingen (1099–1179) reports that valerian is good for relieving gouty pain and stitches in the side; the authors of sixteenth and seventeenth century herbals praised its value as a treatment for difficulty in breathing, weak sight, headaches, coughs, and stab wounds. No word is found there of its calmative and sedative effects. Were these problems unknown at that time? That is scarcely credible, for neither Greek and Roman times nor the Middle Ages were peaceful and tranquil. Nevertheless, the calmative effect of valerian was not discovered until the nineteenth century. Since that time this medicinal plant, in medicine and folk medicine alike, has been considered one of the best calmatives and sedatives.

Valerian, which botanists call *Valeriana officinalis*, has many common names, including garden heliotrope, all-heal, English valerian, German valerian, great wild valerian, vandalroot, phu, setwall, amantilla, nard, and cat's love. In Switzerland and many places in central Baden, Germany, it also is known as Denemarcha (Abbess Hildegard of Bingen also

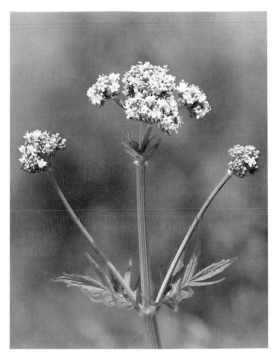

Valerian

used that name) or Dammarg. The origin of this name cannot be explained with certainty; we suppose that the medieval herb sellers dealt in valerian under the name of "Danish root," giving it a foreign name to increase its value.

Valerian grows in damp meadows as well as in dry habitats—from the lowlands to the mountains. This vigorous perennial grows more than 39 inches (1 m) tall. The stem, on which large, feathery, unpaired leaves grow in an opposite arrangement, is squared and hollow. The small reddish-white flowers, which bloom in the months of June, July, and August, grow in clusters (umbels) at the ends of the stems. A number of subspecies and varieties of valerian grow in this country; they differ in the color of the flowers (some darker, some lighter, ranging to pure white) and the number of the pinnules, or feathery leaves (some have only 11, others as many as 21).

Valerian is cultivated for medicinal use. From its root (rhizome), various preparations are derived: a tea, a tincture (*Valerianae tinctura = Tinctura Valerianae*), and valerian baths.

The German Office of Health confirms that valerian has an effect on states of nervous excitement, insomnia, and cramplike pain of nervous origin affecting the stomach and intestinal areas. To that I would like to add: It also is effective in treating cardiac and circulatory disorders of nervous origin.

Cultivation

Valerian grows well in a fairly large garden. It can be started from seed, but it is simpler to buy a few plants at a garden store. Plant valerian in a sunny or partially shady location and keep it damp at all times, because without moisture it will not develop vigorous roots. The soil should be limy. Set the plants 12 to 16 inches (30–40 cm) apart.

You can also grow valerian in limy garden soil in tubs, for your balcony or patio—primarily as an ornamental, however, because valerian is a stately, handsome plant. Please water well in this case also.

If you raise valerian for the sake of its medicinally useful roots, however, you will have to cut off the flowering shoots so that the roots can develop well. After only one year you can harvest the valerian roots. After digging up and washing the plants, hang them up in bunches to dry (see Proper Harvesting and Careful Preparation, page 138).

Wild Strawberry: Almost Nothing Is More Delicious

All the cultivars and breeds, the many strains of strawberries available for sale to us, rank far behind the tiny wild strawberry in terms of both taste and vitamin and mineral content.

It is no surprise, then, that medicine makes use of the wild strawberry. More precisely, "folk medicine," rather than medicine, because despite reports from clinical sources confirming that fresh wild strawberries improve liver and gallbladder function and that "strawberry days" (4.4 ounces [125 g] of wild strawberries eaten three times a day, one or two days a week) help

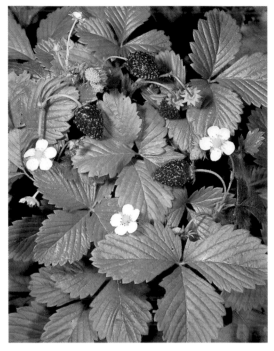

Wild Strawberry

protect the liver, a physician will hardly prescribe them.

Wild strawberry leaves contain large amounts of tannin, have a mildly antidiarrheal effect, and for this reason are admirably suited as an ingredient of a house tea or of tea blends used to treat rheumatism, gout, and metabolic disorders.

Fragaria vesca is the botanical name of the wild strawberry, which belongs to the rose family (Rosaceae). It grows on embankments, along the edges of forest paths, in clearings, and in sunny glades   in flat land and on up to the tree line in the mountains. Even today it still is quite common, although—regrettably for would-be gatherers—large numbers of wild strawberries rarely cover sizable areas any more.

This rosette plant produces long runners, which creep over the ground and take root at the nodes. Wild strawberries reach a height of 2 to 8 inches (5–20 cm). The leaves are long-stalked, and each leaf consists of three leaflets. The upper surfaces of the leaves are light green, the undersides, whitish to gray-green and hairy. The flowers consist of five white petals, five green sepals, and an outer calyx. After the flowers fade, the flower receptacles become fleshy and enlarge to form accessory fruits, which we know as strawberries. The tiny, hard-shelled, shiny nucules (fruitlets) are embedded in the accessory fruit. Wild strawberries bloom from May to June.

Cultivation

It is senseless to plan to introduce wild strawberries into your garden of medicinal or culinary herbs. They would do poorly there and produce almost no fruits. If you have a park, however, and can offer the wild strawberry its natural living conditions, you should try to set out a few small plants there. The runners that have taken root are set in the early summer; if the environment suits the plant, it will grow well.

Willow Bark: Long Forgotten—in Demand Again Today

Before aspirin existed, it was the active substances of willow bark (aspirin-like compounds) that were used to treat fever, headache, and rheumatic pain. In addition, willow bark was an integral component of various tea blends. Then, however, when people no longer had to rely on the salicin and salicylic esters and glucosides of willow bark because acetylsalicylic acid could be produced so easily and cheaply, willow bark was forgotten as a remedy for fever, pain, and rheumatism. Today, as more and more people are recalling the value of natural remedies, willow bark once again serves to allay fever and pain.

Please note
The active substances, however, may irritate the mucous membranes of the stomach, and for this reason people with sensitive stomachs should refrain from drinking willow bark tea.

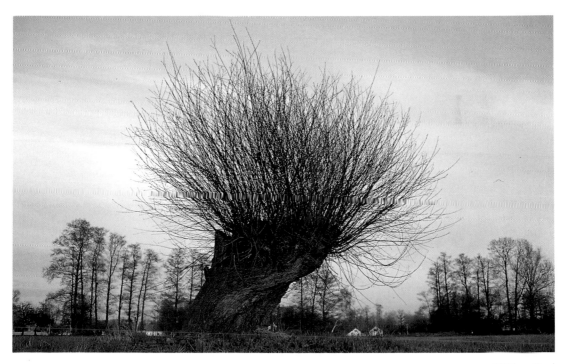

Willow Bark

The German Office of Health validates the efficacy of willow bark in treating feverish diseases, headaches, and rheumatic ailments.

The tea drug is peeled in spring from moderately large branches and dried. The bark comes from various willow species, including the white willow (*Salix alba* L.), purple willow (*Salix purpurea* L.), basket willow, or osier (*Salix daphnoides* L.), and brittle willow, or withy (*Salix fragilis* L.).

Cultivation

Unless your property is extensive, raising willow in your garden is not recommended.

Wormwood: A Boon for the Stomach

"Medicine has to taste bitter; otherwise, it's no good." This old folk wisdom applies here, too, in the truest sense of the word, particularly when we think of the great number of ailments that affect the gastrointestinal area, as well as those in the gallbladder region. Here it is the bitter constituents that bring about an increase in the production of gastric juice, which more often than not relieves the problems. People who cannot easily digest the food they eat, who after eating complain of a feeling of fullness, flatulence, or pain from pressure, whose meal lies heavily on their stomach, and who have no appetite find relief in drinking bitter tea, particularly wormwood tea. It also has become apparent that people who have gallstones can ward off colic by promptly sipping a cup of very warm wormwood tea. In addition to the bitter constituents, the essential oil has a role to play in the effect.

The German Office of Health is somewhat more reserved in assessing this efficacious medicinal plant, particularly where the prevention of colic in people with gallstones is concerned. This probably is due only to the fact that more recent studies are not yet available. As for the curative effect on stomach ailments, however, wormwood finds approval there as well. The following appears on the package circular of the standard permit under the heading

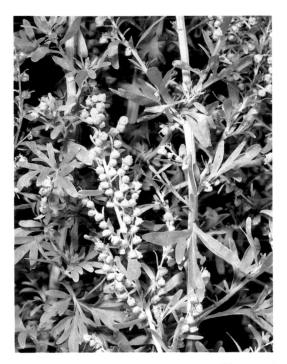

Wormwood

"Application": For stomach ailments due, for example, to insufficient production of gastric juice; for stimulating the appetite. Gastric and duodenal ulcers are listed as contraindications.

Wormwood (as well as its milder "brother," mugwort; see page 190) also has importance as a seasoning for fatty foods such as roast goose and duck, fried potatoes, fatty pork roasts, and fatty sausages. With goose and duck it is added to the stuffing. Alternatively, some wormwood can be placed in the roasting pan. Apart from that, powdered wormwood also can be used for flavoring dishes before or after they are cooked.

Wormwood, known to botanists as *Artemisia absinthium,* belongs to the composite family (Asteraceae = Compositae). It is also known by the common names of absinthe, absinthium, green ginger, madderwort, and old woman.

Wormwood is a perennial herbaceous plant that reaches a height of 24 to more than 39 inches (60 cm–1 m). Wormwood grows erect and branched. Both the stem and the leaves are covered with a coat of silvery gray hair, which lends the entire plant a gray luster. This also clearly distinguishes wormwood from mugwort, the stem of which is tinged with reddish brown. Wormwood leaves are tripinnatifid, large at the bottom of the plant and smaller toward the top, where they also are "more simply" formed. The peduncle bears a great many hemispherical, nodding, light-yellow tiny flower heads (mugwort flowers are usually reddish), arranged in freely flowering branched panicles. The entire plant has a strong, biting smell.

Both wormwood and mugwort like sunny locations along roadsides, river banks, and fences, mugwort, however, is more common there.

Cultivation

This herbaceous perennial can be grown in tubs on your patio or in your garden in sunny places. It is easiest to get finished plants in a garden store.

Wormwood flourishes best in limy, nutritious soils. Nitrogenous fertilizer will ensure that the shoots do not lignify too heavily. The best time for planting is fall. If you have acquired a large plant, cut it back, as this stimulates it to "shoot" luxuriantly the next spring. Every three to five years you need to divide the stems that are in the process of shooting forth and transplant them.

The parts harvested are the flower-bearing terminal and lateral shoots. Tie them into bunches, dry them in the open air, then store them in a dry, dark place.

To use as a seasoning that will strengthen the stomach, add a small piece of shoot to dishes during preparation. It can be removed easily once the food is cooked. Primarily the leaves and the shoot tips are used in making tea.

Yarrow: The Vulnerary Herb of Achilles

Botanists know yarrow as *Achillea millefolium.* It has numerous common names, including bloodwort, milfoil, nosebleed, old man's pepper, sanguinary, soldier's woundwort, stanchgrass, and thousand-leaf. Yarrow grows in meadows,

along roadsides, on embankments, and in landfills and garbage dumps. In folk medicine yarrow has quite a broad range of applications. Foremost among them is the treatment of gastrointestinal and gallbladder complaints, lack of appetite, and catarrhs of the digestive organs. These fields of application are acknowledged by the German Office of Health. This medicinal plant is just as effective in the treatment of nervousness and sleep disturbances, because the substances contained in yarrow help to produce a feeling of peace and relaxation, particularly in women going through menopause. A great many tea blends used to relieve these complaints contain yarrow as a supplementary component. Yarrow, either as a tea or as a bath additive, has proved helpful in allaying rheumatic pain.

In antiquity and during the Middle Ages, yarrow was used primarily to treat wounds. According to legend, the Greek hero Achilles was taught by the centaur Chiron to use yarrow as a treatment for battle wounds.

Yarrow grows from 8 to 18 inches (20–45 cm), sometimes to 24 inches (60 cm), tall. It is

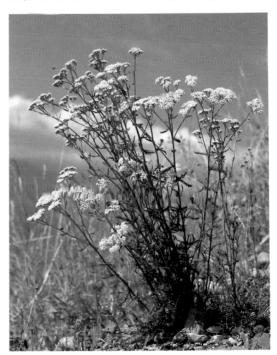

Yarrow

identifiable in part by the finely divided leaves (*millefolium* = "of a thousand leaves") and the erect flowering stalk with the white or reddish composite flowers that are arranged in panicled false umbels, and in part by its aromatic scent, which is released when the leaves and flowers are crushed between one's fingers.

Please note

Small numbers of people have an allergic reaction upon contact with the plant; their skin turns red and an itchy rash develops. Such people also cannot tolerate yarrow tea or yarrow baths. Discontinue the treatment at once if problems of this kind appear. Then the allergic reaction will disappear quickly.

Cultivation

In our great-grandmothers' day, yarrow grew in every herb garden. If we want to do things our great-grandmothers' way, we should bring a few small plants home from the meadow or from a nursery in early spring: Raising them from seed is possible, of course, but quite involved. Set the plants 6 to 8 inches (15–20 cm) apart in normal garden soil in a sunny location. Everything else will take care of itself, if you ensure that the location is free from standing water. Yarrow, a herbaceous perennial, "shoots" anew year after year; to propagate it in your garden, divide the stems in fall and move them to new locations.

For medicinal purposes, all the flowering parts above the ground are used, everything except the lower, lignified parts of the plant. Cut the plant a handsbreadth above the ground, hang it up to dry in the open air, then cut it into small pieces and store it in containers that can be tightly closed, protected from light and dampness.

Appendix

Using Healing Plants Properly

Most of the medicinal plant applications recommended in this guide involve the use of teas. The teas may be applied both internally and externally.

Internal application—drinking the tea—is the best-known and most common form of application. If an internally applied tea made from a medicinal plant is to develop its full effect, it is essential that you follow to the letter all instructions regarding the amount of the drug to be used, the length of steeping, the temperature of the water used in preparing the tea, and the manner in which the tea is to be drunk—in sips, cold, warm, or hot.

The term *external application* refers to the use of a tea—particularly a tea brewed from a single drug, not a blend—in full or partial baths, progressively hot footbaths, inhalations, steam baths, or washes; in the treatment of wounds; or as a gargle or a mouthwash. Here, too, the guidelines given for preparation and application need to be followed exactly. For most of the medicinal plant teas recommended here, there is a standard method of preparation and application. If no other directions accompany the recommendations in the individual chapters, the following instructions apply.

Instructions for Preparing and Applying the Teas

Internal Application

● **Drinking tea:**
Preparation: Pour 8 ounces (1/4 L) of boiling water over 2 heaping teaspoonfuls of the drug (a single tea or a tea blend), let steep, covered, for ten minutes, then strain through a sieve.

Application: In sips, drink two to three cups of tea, moderately warm, between meals. Sweeten with honey to taste (diabetics do not sweeten!).

External Applications

● **Full baths:**
Preparation: If you use ready-made extracts from the pharmacy, follow the directions for preparation given on the package. Alternatively, follow the directions in this book to prepare the extract yourself.

Application: Full baths with drug extracts are taken in a bathtub at temperatures between 95 and 100°F (35–38°C). The bath should last 10 to 15 minutes. It is advisable to rest in bed immediately afterward, because the warmth of the bed and peace and quiet will intensify the effect of the bath.

● **Partial baths**
Have a washbasin or a small tub ready.
Preparation: Use 1 tablespoonful of the recommended drug per quart (1 L) of liquid. Pour cold water over the drug, bring to a boil, let steep for ten minutes, strain, and let cool to a temperature of 95 to 104°F (35–40°C).

Application: Put this mixture in the basin or tub and soak the diseased or injured body parts (finger, hand, foot) in it at the given temperature (95-104°F [35–40°C]) for about ten minutes, then dry and cover the parts.

● **Progressively hot foot baths:**
Have a pot and a deep footbath ready. For the recommended footbath, use a mixture of thyme tea and horsetail tea.

Preparation: Prepare 1 quart (1 L) of thyme tea and 1 pint (1/2 L) of horsetail tea in a pot—pour boiling water over 4 tablespoonfuls of the aerial parts of thyme and 2 tablespoonfuls of the aerial parts of horsetail, let steep, covered, for ten minutes, then strain through a sieve. Put this mixture into the footbath.

Application: Begin the footbath in 98.6°F (37°C) water, then, by adding hot water, slowly increase the temperature as long as it is bearable. End the footbath after 10 to 15 minutes, dry your feet, and put on warm socks.

● **Inhalations, steam baths**
Get a suitable container ready, along with cloths or large bath towels for covering.

Preparation: Put one small handful of the recommended drugs in the container and pour 1 pint to 1 quart (1/2–1 L) of boiling water over them.

Application of the inhalation: Cover your head and the container with a cloth, then slowly and deeply inhale the herbal vapors through your mouth and/or nose.

Application of the steam bath: Let the vapors act on your skin. For steam baths in the anal and genital area, put 3 quarts (3 L) of hot water with 3 to 4 tablespoonfuls of the drug in a sturdy container and sit on it.

Once the steam has ceased to rise, reheat the mixture by adding hot water—the application should last five to ten minutes.

● **Damp dressings, compresses**
Get cotton pads, gauze pads, and bandaging material ready.

Preparation: Prepare the recommended tea according to the directions in this book.

Application: Soak the cotton pad or gauze pad in the tea, squeeze it out slightly, lay it on the areas to be treated, and secure it with a bandage or a compress. The bandage/compress should remain in place for several hours. When it is dry, dampen it several times with whatever

tea you are using; it does not need to be replaced.

● **Gargle, mouthwash**
Preparation: Prepare the recommended tea according to the directions in this book and let it cool to a temperature that you can tolerate.

Application: Gargle with the (unsweetened) tea in mouthfuls. It is important that the actual gargling (minus the necessary interruptions) last at least one minute. The mouthwash should spend a total of about five minutes in your mouth.

● **Little herbal bags**
Preparation: Put the recommended drug blend into a small cotton or linen bag. Place the bag in boiling-hot water for about ten minutes, take it out, lay it between two small boards, and press them together firmly to squeeze the water out. Then let the bag cool to whatever temperature the patient finds tolerable (please test this in advance, to avoid burns).

On page 46 an alternative method of preparation is described.

Application: Lay the bag, which should be quite warm, on the affected area.

Herbal pillow: This application entails the placement of a small bag—dry—filled with the recommended blend of drugs under your pillow at night.

Photos:
de Cuveland: 172. Eisenbeiss: 4, 110, 126, 170, 209. Eigstler: 141, 148, 157, 197, 213. Fischer: inside back cover, 2 and 4. Greiner & Mayer: 88. Hagen: 139. König: 19, 156, 161, 196. Photo-Center: 28, 160, 187, 210. Reinhard: inside back cover, 1; 53, 102, 136, 164, 169, 171, 174, 178, 181, 190, 199, 202, 206. Reuter: 144, 151, 168, 183, 189, 193, 204. Riedmiller: 145, 163, 211; back cover. Schacht: 146. Scherz: title page; 40, 68, 147, 154, 164, 165, 173, 177, 184, 191, 192, 194, 198, 205. Schimmitat: 140, 150, 152, 162, 166, 175, 185, 208. Schrempp: 82, 132, 155, 157, 167, 179, 180, 186, 207. Skogstad: 142, 161. Strauss: 176, 195. Wothe: 153, 188.

Index

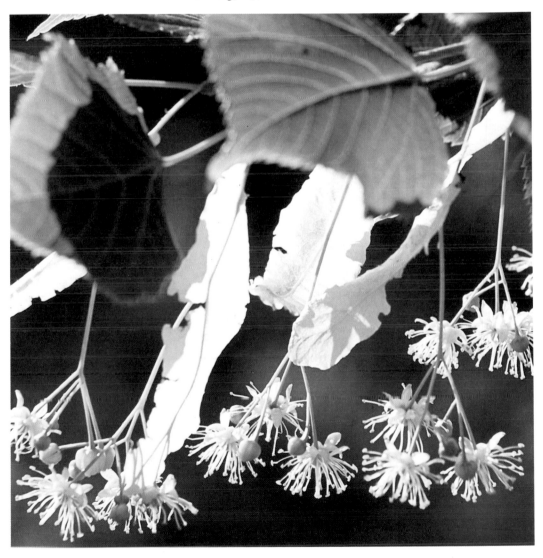

Linden Flowers

Glossary

Accumbent Lying against, facing, or extending up something. Contrast DECUMBENT.

Adventitious Root Root that forms on a stem or leaf after it has been cut and planted. In some cases, the cutting is treated with rooting hormone.

Alterative Medication that gradually overcomes an unhealthy condition.

Amara Term used to designate bitter-constituent drugs. Pure bitters are called *amara tonica*; bitters containing ESSENTIAL OILS are called *amara aromatica*; bitters containing acrid substances are called *amara acria*.

Antispasmodic Medication that relieves muscular cramps or spasms.

Aperitive Medication that has a gentle, laxative effect.

Axil Upper angle between a leaf and a stem; usually contains an axillary bud.

Bract Leaf that forms from an AXIL, often associated with an INFLORESCENCE.

Calmative Medication that reduces nervousness or excitement. Also called a *sedative* or *tranquilizer*.

Carminative Medication that aids in the expulsion of intestinal gases, or that reduces their formation.

Choleretic Medication that increases bile flow.

Corolla Collective term for the petals that are the second whorl of the floral envelopes. It is interior to the SEPALS.

Corona Crown; any appendage that stands between the COROLLA and the STAMENS.

Crenate With rounded teeth along the margin. Contrast SERRATE.

Cuspidate With an apex abruptly and concavely constricted into an elongated, pointed tip.

Decumbent Lying down or along the ground. Contrast ACCUMBENT.

Decussate Arranged oppositely in pairs along a stem. Each successive pair is set at right angles to the preceding pair, producing four distinct rows of leaves.

Dehiscent Fruit that splits open at maturity, releasing or exposing its contents.

Dioecious Species that has male and female flowers growing on different plants. Contrast MONOECILOUS.

Diuretic Medication that increases the production and flow of urine.

Drupe Stone fruit. An outer fleshy layer covers an interior stony or woody core containing a single seed, as in the cherry or peach.

Electuary Medication that has been sweetened—usually with sugar or honey.

Embrocation Liquid medication that is applied to the skin to relieve pain or inflammation.

Essential Oil Highly volatile oils found in most plants. Also called *ethereal oils*.

Flavonoids Collective term for substances found in plants. Typical uses include as a diuretic, an antispasmodic, and for the relief of certain cardiac and circulatory disorders.

Glume Small chafflike BRACT found at the base of the flower pairs of most grass. The chaff of cereal grains.

Glycosides Widely distributed plant substances that consist of a sugar and a non-sugar portion. The non-sugar (aglycone) is largely responsible for the medicinal effect.

Imparpinnate Odd PINNATE; a pinnately compound leaf with a terminal leaflet.

Inflorescence Cluster of flowers.

Involucral BRACTS subtending an INFLORESCENCE.

Lanceolate Lance-shaped; a leaf much longer than wide and gradually tapering from below the middle to the apex.

Leukorrhea Whitish vaginal discharge, which may be caused by bacteria, fungi, trichomonads, or constitutional factors.

Lignify To become woody by thickening cell walls with lignin.

Ligule Little tongue; applied to the small appendage on the upper side of the leaf of grasses at the junction of the sheath and blade. Also used for the strap-shaped COROLLA of the circumferential flowers of the INFLORESCENCE of the aster or sunflower family (Asteraceae).

Mesocarp Middle layer of a fruit. It may be fleshy as in DRUPE or woody as in nuts.

Monoecious Species in which male and female flowers grow on the same plant. Contrast DIOECIOUS.

Mucolytic Causing mucus to break down into a more watery liquid.

Mucilage Plant substance that expands greatly when mixed with water, producing a viscous liquid that can coat mucous membranes.

Myocardial infarction Deterioration of part of the muscular wall of the heart caused by inadequate blood supply (usually resulting from a clot or embolism). A *heart attack*.

Neurodystonia Nervous debility and exhaustion. Symptoms include palpitations, anxiety, dizziness, headaches, clammy hands and feet. An older term for this condition is *neurasthenia*.

Obovate Oval that is widest in the upper half. Contrast OVATE.

Ovate Oval that is widest in the lower half (as in a hen's egg). Contrast OBOVATE.

Panicle Pyramidal INFLORESCENCE formed by multiple branches. Each branch is a RACEME.

Papilionaceous Flower form thought to resemble a butterfly.

Peduncle Stalk of an INFLORESCENCE or of a flower when borne singly.

Pharmacognocy Study of medicinal plants.

Phyllary Individual INVOLUCRAL BRACT.

Phytotherapy Therapeutic use of medicinal plants.

Pinnate Leaves arranged on opposite sides of a stem.

Pistil Female flower part that bears the STIGMA.

Pruinous (also prunose) Having a waxy layer or bloom on the surface (as in a prune).

Pseudocarp False fruit.

Quinquefid Five parted.

Raceme Form of INFLORESCENCE with several single flowers growing on individual small stems and along a larger main stem.

Refrigerant Medication that reduces bodily temperature.

Rhizome Underground horizontal stem with scale leaves at the nodes that bears shoots above and roots below.

Saponin Plant extract that produces soapy bubbles when mixed with water. Saponins can emulsify oils and cause thick mucous to liquify.

Sepals Outermost floral whorl that serves as a protective enclosure for the petals (COROLLA), STAMENS, and young fruit.

Serrate Toothed along the margin with sharp, forward pointing teeth. Contrast CRENATE.

Silicic acid Substance that plants absorb from the soil. Horsetail, borage, and grasses are high in silicic acid.

Spasmolytic Medication that relieves muscular cramps or spasms.

Spatulate Spoon-shaped; rounded above and constricted below.

Squarrose Abruptly spreading or recurved above the base.

Stamen Pollen-bearing male organ of the flower.

Stigma Part of the PISTIL that receives pollen.

Stolon Above ground or underground side shoots that grow from the base of the stem, the flower rosette, the mother plant, or the root crown. Also called a *runner*.

Stomachic Medication that stimulates the appetite.

Stypic Medication that helps stop the flow of blood from a wound.

Sudorific Medication that increases perspiration.

Syncarp A multiple or aggregate fleshy fruit as in the mulberry or blackberry.

Tannin Plant substances that are able to bind proteins of the skin, transforming them into resistant, insoluble substances.

Trichomonad Parasitic protozoan that sometimes infects the genitals.

Umbel INFLORESCENCE in which the PEDUNCLE or pedicels of a flower cluster arise from a common point.

Vulnerary Medication that is applied to open wounds to aid in healing.

Sources

Sources of Herbs

Golden Earth Herbs
Box 2
Torreon, NM 87061
USA
505/384-2916

Haussmann's Pharmacy, Inc.
534-536 W. Girard Avenue
Philadelphia, PA 19123
USA
215/627-2143

Herbalist & Alchemist
P.O. Box 458
Bloomsbury, NJ 08804-0458
USA
908/479-6679

The Herb Shed
51 Scotts Landing Road
Southampton, NY 11968
USA
516/283-6139

The Herb Works
180 Southgate Drive #5
Guelph, ON N1G 4P5
Canada
519/824-4280

Indiana Botanic Garden
P.O. Box 5
Hammond, IN 46325
USA
219/947-4040

L.H. Vitamins
37-10 Crescent Street
Long Island City, NY 11101
USA
516/231-5522

Nature's Herb Company
Box 118, Dept. 34, Q
Norway, IA 52318
USA
800/365-4372

Neal's Yard Remedies
2 Neal's Yard
Covent Garden
London WC2
England
071/284039

Pacific Botanicals
4350 Fish Hatchery Road
Grants Pass, OR 97527
USA
503/479-7777

Rainbow Light
207 McPherson Street
Santa Cruz, CA 95060
USA
In CA: 800/227-0555
Elsewhere: 800/635-1233

Yerba Prima
P.O. Box 5009
Berkeley, CA 94705
USA
415/632-7477

Note: Several of the companies listed above also supply herbal preparations, including tinctures, salves, and encapsulated products.

Sources of Herb Seeds

W. Atlee Burpee Company
300 Park Avenue
Warminster, PA 18774
USA
215/674-4900

William Dam Seeds
Box 8400, 279 Highway 8
Dundas, ON L9H 6M1
Canada
416/628 6641

Exotica Seed Company
P.O. Box 160
Vista, CA 92805
USA
619/724-9093

George W. Park Seed Company
Cokesbury Road
Greenwood, SC 29647-0001
USA
800/845-3369

Richter's
Canada Herb Specialists
357 Highway 47
Goodwood, ON L0C 1A0
Canada
416/640-6677

Shepherd's Garden Seeds
6116 Highway 9
Felton, CA 95018
USA
408/335-6910

Stokes Seeds, Inc.
P.O. Box 548
Buffalo, NY 14240
USA
416/688-4300

Sutton Seeds
Hele Road
Torquay
Devon TQ2 7QJ
England
803/612011

Sources of Information

The American Botanical Council
P.O. Box 201660
Austin, TX 78720
USA

American Herb Association
P.O. Box 1673
Nevada City, CA 95959
USA

Herb Research Foundation
1007 Pearl Street
Suite 200
Boulder, CO 80303
USA

Note: The lists of Sources and Publications were compiled with the assistance of the Herb Research Foundation. Addresses and phone numbers were verified immediately prior to publication, but may have changed since.

For Further Reading

Books

Budavari, S. ed. *Merck Index, 11th ed.* Rahway, New Jersey: Merck & Co., 1989.

Duke, J. A. *Handbook of Medicinal Herbs.* Boca Raton, Florida: CRC Press, 1985.

Jarvis, D. C. *Folk Medicine.* Philadelphia: W.H. Allen & Co., 1960.

Kingsbury, J. M. *Poisonous Plants of the United States and Canada.* Englewood Cliffs, New Jersey: Prentice-Hall, 1964.

Kreig, M. B. *Green Medicine.* Skokie, Illinois: Rand McNally, 1964.

Lewis, W. H., and M. P. F. Elvin-Lewis. *Medical Botany: Plants Affecting Man's Health.* New York: John Wiley & Sons, 1977.

Lucas, R. *Nature's Medicines.* New York: Universal-Award House, 1966.

Marks, G., and W. K. Beatly. *The Medical Garden.* New York: Charles Scribner's & Sons, 1971.

McRae, Bobbi A. *The Herb Companion: Wishbook and Resource Guide.* Loveland, Colorado: Interweave Press, 1992.

Orbell, A. *A Compendium of Botanical Remedies: Physiomedical Practice.* Exeter, England: Ilford, 1967.

Vogel, V.J. *American Indian Medicine.* Norman, Oklahoma: University of Oklahoma Press, 1970.

Publications

Foster's Botanical and Herb Review (quarterly)
P.O. Box 106
Eureka Springs, AR 72632   501/253-7309

Herbalgram (quarterly)
Subscription available through the American Herb Association or the Herbal Research Foundation (see page 223.)

The Herb Companion (bi-monthly)
Interweave Press
201 East 4th Street
Loveland, CO 80537   303/669-7672

The Herb Quarterly
P.O. Box 689
San Anselmo, CA 94960   415/455-9540

Acknowlegements

We gratefully acknowledge the assistance of the following:

Dennis Stevenson, Ph.D., Director of the Harding Laboratory of the New York Botanical Garden, acted as Consulting Editor of this edition.

Florence H. Segelman, Ph.D. pharmacognocist, served as adviser regarding the therapeutic use of the remedies and their consistency with current American health practices.

The Herb Research Foundation, an independent, nonprofit educational and research organization assisted in the compilation of the lists of Sources and Publications.

The Author

Mannfried Pahlow has a degree in pharmacy. He is the author of books for a specialized audience, as well as for the general public. He is a member of the Society for Phytotherapy, and in 1963 he was awarded the Serturn Medal.

Library of Congress Catalog Card No. 92-45671
International Standard Book No. 0-8120-1498-7

Library of Congress Cataloging-in-Publication Data

Pahlow, Mannfried.
    [Heilpflanzen. English]
    The healing plants : self-treatment of the most common everyday complaints and disorders with selected medicinal plants : time-tested recipes for teas, tea blends, tinctures, ointments, inhalations, compresses, and baths: expert advice and dependable remedies : Mannfried Pahlow : consulting editor, Dennis W. Stevenson : [translated from the German by Kathleen Luft].
    Includes bibliographical references and index.
    ISBN 0-8120-1498-7
    1. Herbs—Therapeutic use. 2. Medicinal plants. 3. Materia medica, Vegetable. I. Stevenson, Dennis W. II. Title.
    RM666.H33P313 1993   92-45671
    615'.321—dc20   CIP

PRINTED IN HONG KONG
3456 9927 98765432